# RESEARCHING FOOD HABITS

# THE ANTHROPOLOGY OF FOOD AND NUTRITION

General Editor: *Helen Macbeth*

# RESEARCHING FOOD HABITS

*Methods and Problems*

*Edited by*

Helen Macbeth and Jeremy MacClancy

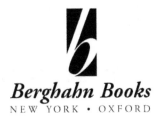

*Berghahn Books*
NEW YORK • OXFORD

First published in 2004 by

*Berghahn Books*
www.berghahnbooks.com

**Library of Congress Cataloging-in-Publication Data**

Researching food habits : methods and problems / edited by Helen Macbeth and
Jeremy MacClancy.
    p. cm. -- (The anthropology of food and nutrition ; v. 5)
    Includes bibliographical references and index.
    ISBN 978-1-57181-544-6 (hardback : alk.paper) -- ISBN 978-1-57181-545-3 (pbk. :
alk. paper)
    1. Food habits. 2. Food preferences. I. Macbeth, Helen M. II. MacClancy, Jeremy.
    III. Series

GT2850.R47 2003
394.1'2--dc22

                                                                    2003063589


**British Library Cataloguing in Publication Data**

A catalogue record for this book is available from the British Library

Printed in the United States on acid-free paper

ISBN 978-1-57181-544-6 hardback
ISBN 978-1-57181-545-3 paperback

# CONTENTS

# LIST OF FIGURES

# LIST OF TABLES

# PREFACE

This book is about research techniques. It is a 'how-to-do-it' book for the new researcher or student who intends to undertake research in the 'anthropology of food'. The phrase, the anthropology of food, has become an accepted abbreviation for the study of anthropological perspectives on food, diet and nutrition. It has immediately to be said, however, that there are many aspects of anthropology and many ways to be interested in the topic of human food. Researchers who wish to gain a holistic understanding of almost any topic regarding human food, frequently feel virtually obliged to use a variety of research methods. They feel this sense of obligation for two main reasons: (1) because the anthropology of food encompasses so many perspectives, and (2) because these perspectives often interrelate in a significant manner. Within this book, the relevance and history of a variety of academic approaches to the anthropology of food are discussed and both their diversity and their modes of interaction are emphasised. Up until the publication of this book, these different approaches, and therefore any information on appropriate research methods, were only to be found under different, separate disciplinary classifications in any library. For all these reasons, members of the International Commission on the Anthropology of Food (ICAF) thought it worthwhile to edit a book which brought together into one volume a cross-disciplinary selection of relevant research methods.

An immediate question at this initial stage has to be: 'Who does what? Which kind of food anthropologist tends to follow, conventionally, which kind of approach and how, at the simplest level, do these approaches overlap?' Nutritionists, human biologists and biological anthropologists study food items and their chemical constituents in order to understand the biochemical effects of these foods on human physiology, health, behaviour, survival and fertility. Yet, they also need to know whether any food items under consideration are consumed by the people they are studying and in what quantities. A broad range of human attitudes to those food items has an overwhelming effect on whether the items will be consumed, in what form, to what extent and whether they are even available and affordable. These attitudes in turn vary with social, cultural and economic patterns and situations, which are studied by social scientists, especially by social anthropologists, social psychologists and market economists, and yet they should not be ignored by the biologists. At the same time, those concerned with the social significance of different consumption patterns should bear in mind that the food and drink items do have nutritive significance. They should also recognise the value of their information to the nutritionists and dieticians, and vice versa.

Recognition of this multiplicity of interconnecting perspectives is essential for students and researchers working on the anthropology of food. However, it is hard to find guidance on how to pursue cross-disciplinary research when academic guidance traditionally comes only from each specialism separately. One aim of this volume is to aid new researchers in their choice of which methods can best answer cross-disciplinary questions. There are currently no research methods that should be considered specific only to the anthropology of food, and many anthropologists of food have had to adapt methods from other disciplines. In the twenty-first century we are still on a relatively new journey in finding out how to coordinate multidisciplinary research, but in this volume diverse approaches are introduced, although because of space some perspectives have not been covered. The contributors are specialists from very different sub-disciplines within anthropology, and so, inevitably, there is only tenuous linkage between some chapters. The objective of the editors has not been to integrate these into some *one* anthropological approach, which does not and cannot exist, but to place at the disposal of the prospective researcher a range of methods in adjacent chapters. Researcher-readers are invited to 'pick and mix' in order to put together, for their own specific purposes, novel cross-disciplinary conjunctions of the established methods.

The difference between 'quantitative data' and 'qualitative data' should be explained at the outset. Quantitative data are data that can be enumerated. This is obvious for measurements, whether of units consumed, of chemical constituents, of calories contained, of biomedical characteristics or of the number of consumers themselves. However, a numerical approach can also be used when non-numerical information is converted to numbers. This can, for example, be when the intensity of response or feeling is recorded on a numerical scale or when non-numerical information is coded into numbers, usually ordinal numbers, either by a respondent choosing options or by a researcher entering data on to a computer. In contrast, qualitative data are information that has not been converted into numbers. The data are descriptive and sensitive to much subtler levels of variation than can be reduced to numbers. A far richer insight is gained from conversations, open-ended interviews and participant observation than can be constrained into data appropriate for numerical analysis. However, qualitative data are harder to analyse or compare objectively and there is often a greater element of a researcher's subjective conclusions in the results.

It is incorrect to assume that the division between numerate and non-numerate analysis corresponds to a division between social and biological sciences. It is true that most social anthropologists are primarily concerned with qualitative data, and so are not generally required to have the basic grounding in statistics that is necessary for those in other social sciences, such as social psychology, economics and sociology. It is also true, however, that while a great deal of biological research is based on statistical material, not all is. In reviewing the methods described in this book the new researcher should note where the contributors recommend a more qualitative or a more quantitative approach, or a combination of qualitative and quantitative methods.

The editors are most grateful to the contributors, without whose work and willingness to cooperate this book would not have been possible. ICAF(UK) is thanked for their support of the meeting which brought these contributors together. Finally, we are grateful to Jennifer Jay for assistance with the index and to Annie Merselis for clerical work on early drafts.

*H.M.M. and J.V.M.*
*March 2003*

# LIST OF CONTRIBUTORS

**Dr Igor de Garine**

Centre National de la Recherche Scientifique, Paris, France.

**Dra. Isabel González Turmo**

Departamento de Antropología Social, Universidad de Sevilla, Seville, Spain.

**Professor C. Jeya K. Henry**

Department of Nutrition, School of Biological and Molecular Sciences, Oxford Brookes University, Oxford, United Kingdom.

**Dr Claude Marcel Hladik**

Centre National de la Recherche Scientifique, Museum National d'Histoire Naturelle, Brunoy, France.

**Dr Annie Hubert**

Centre Nationale de la Recherche Scientifique, Université de la Méditerranée, Marseille, France.

**Dr Helen M. Macbeth**

Anthropology Department, School of Social Sciences and Law, Oxford Brookes University, Oxford, United Kingdom.

**Professor Jeremy V. MacClancy**

Anthropology Department, School of Social Sciences and Law, Oxford Brookes University, Oxford, United Kingdom.

**Dr Gerald Mars**

The Newcastle Business School and The London Metropolitan University, London, United Kingdom.

**Dr Valerie Mars**

Social historian, London, United Kingdom.

| | |
|---|---|
| **Prof. Catedrático José Mataix Verdú** | Departamento de Fisiología and El Instituto de Nutrición y Tecnología de Alimentos, Universidad de Granada, Granada, Spain. |
| **Dr F. Xavier Medina** | European Institute of the Mediterranean, Barcelona, Spain. |
| **Dr Ellen Messer** | Friedman School of Nutrition Science and Policy, Tufts University, Boston, United States. |
| **Fiona Mowatt** | Anthropology Department, School of Social Sciences and Law, Oxford Brookes University, Oxford, United Kingdom. |
| **Dr Patrick Pasquet** | Eco-Anthropologie et Etnobiologie, Museé de l'Homme, Paris, France. |
| **Dr Nancy J. Pollock** | Anthropology and Development Studies, Victoria University, Wellington, New Zealand. |
| **Dr Bruno Simmen** | Centre National de la Recherche Scientifique, Museum National d'Histoire Naturelle, Brunoy, France. |
| **Professor Attila T. Szabó** | Department of Botany, Institute of Biology, University of Veszprém, Veszprém, Hungary. |
| **Dr Stanley J. Ulijaszek** | Institute of Social and Cultural Anthropology, University of Oxford, Oxford, United Kingdom. |

# INTRODUCTION
## HOW TO DO ANTHROPOLOGIES OF FOOD

*Jeremy MacClancy* and *Helen Macbeth*

Anthropology is a broad school. It always has been. During its emergence in the nineteenth century the umbrella term 'anthropology' sheltered a surprisingly wide range of subjects: from the measuring of people's skulls to see if they were of the criminal types to those campaigning against the evils of slavery. So long as any particular approach embraced the study of humans as social beings it could fit in within the broad rubric of 'anthropology' (from the Greek *anthropos*, human). In this sense anthropology is not so much a discipline, more a loose collection of several different disciplines. Even today the term embraces both laboratory-based molecular geneticists and the most abstracted of social theorists, both those interested in the effect of biological variables within human populations and those researching social dimensions of cognitive processes. In the United States the term has an even broader scope, at times encompassing archaeologists and linguists as well. The leading historian of the subject, George Stocking (2001), has gone so far as to call it the 'boundless discipline'.

Anthropology may indeed be boundless but it has a very dynamic boundlessness. The various disciplines usually grouped within anthropology have come together and moved apart more than once over the course of its history. In particular the physical and the social sides underwent a radical separation from the late-1920s on: the intellectual abuses committed in those times by certain racist anthropologists, especially in Nazi Germany, put many off studying almost any form of physical anthropology for a long period. At much the same time many social anthropologists were keen to establish their own academic distinctiveness and independence (MacClancy 1986, 1995). Despite the exemplary antiracist campaigning of some physical anthropologists who destroyed the scientific credibility of the concept of 'race', it still took several decades for an expanded physical anthropology to regain popularity. By then its leading practitioners had renamed the subject 'biological anthropology',

since it had become more common to study variations within human populations in terms of gene frequencies than in terms of external bodily measurements. It was not until these changes had taken place that significant numbers
of those on either side of the biological/social divide began to consider trying
to work together (Stocking 1988).

In this book we look at one particular sub-section of the almost kaleido-
scopic variety that we call anthropology: the anthropology of food. Its range is
wide, its potential futures even wider and full of promise. However, its history
is surprisingly shallow. We shall sketch it in the briefest manner: de Garine in
his contribution (Chapter One) gives more detail and background.

## The Rises and Fall of Anthropologies of Food

An anthropology of food, recognisable as such, only arose in the 1930s with
the pioneering and exemplary studies of Audrey Richards among the Southern Bantu and the Bemba of Zambia (Richards 1932, 1939). Working within
the strictly functionalist frame created by her supervisor, Malinowski, she
strove to examine the human relationships of a society 'as determined by nutritional needs'; she wanted to 'show how hunger shapes the sentiments which
bind together the members of each social group' (1932: 23). The work of Richards
and her colleagues (e.g., Firth 1934, Fortes and Fortes 1936) dovetailed with
contemporary colonialist concerns about inadequate native diets preventing
locals from joining the labour force.

In North America during this period anthropological studies of food were
conducted by those within the 'culture and personality' school, of which
Margaret Mead was a prominent member. These anthropologists concentrated
on the development of attitudes towards food in different cultures and how
those attitudes affected later social relationships, behaviour and psychosocial
maturation (Messer 1984). In 1940 the United States Government, mindful of
the war and well aware that a significant proportion of its citizens suffered from
nutritional deficiency, established a Committee on Food Habits. The brief
of this interdisciplinary body, whose membership included Mead and Ruth
Benedict, was to study the factors involved in the directed change of food
habits (Freedman 1977). For Mead, the contribution anthropologists could
make towards the problems of dieticians in wartime was (1) to be able to put
food-related activities into their appropriate cultural context, and (2) to provide information about the cultural dynamics underlying social acceptance or
rejection of certain dietary practices (Mead 1943a: 1, see also Mead 1943b;
Guthe and Mead 1945). At the end of the war, the committee was disbanded.
It is curious that anthropologists of the time do not seem to have continued
this style of work. In Britain at least, it appears that in the immediate postwar
decades social anthropologists were usually more interested in developing
anthropological theory than enquiring into what seemed like narrowly practical matters like food (MacClancy 1996).

Interest in the study of food re-emerged most prominently in North America in the mid- to late-1950s as anthropologists such as Julian Steward (1955) and Elman Service (1962) began to propound a cultural ecology. According to this approach, human beings were to be viewed 'as intelligent, technologically equipped and culturally conditioned biological actors existing in open feedback systems with other biological units of their environment. Thus, food becomes a means for the transfer of energy among ecosystem components, and nutritional requirements are conditioned by the multiplicity of ecological factors' (Kandel *et al.* 1980). From the mid-1960s Marvin Harris took on the legacy of this approach, while promoting his own cultural materialism, which proved to be as popular as it was controversial (e.g. Harris 1966, 1979, 1987, Harris and Ross 1987).

The leading opponents of Harris and his followers tended to be structuralists. They were inspired by the work of Claude Lévi-Strauss, who had given the symbolism of food and cooking a primordial position within his vision of the world. The most prominent of these structuralists in the United Kingdom was Mary Douglas, author of the seminal *Purity and Danger* (1966), who was later to co-found the International Commission on the Anthropology of Food. To stereotype slightly, one might say that structuralism tended to attract those who took pleasure in abstracted interpretation and the formal beauty of diagrammatic solutions, while Harris's cultural materialism seemed to appeal to those who saw themselves as more 'down-to-earth' types concerned with supposed facts 'on the ground'. The distance between those interested in either of these approaches was unfortunately exaggerated by the proselytising zeal of their respective advocates. As Messer stated (1984: 212), it was 'a brave soul' who tried to straddle the two.

It was not until the 1980s that social anthropologists of food started to move away from these self-styled polar opposites and to publish sophisticated monographs which were not strictly tied to either structuralist or cultural materialist agendas. Instead, quite simply, the best among them were exemplars of a discriminating eclecticism. The key texts here are above all Sidney Mintz's *Sweetness and Power* (1985), and Mary Weismantel's *Food, Gender and Poverty in the Ecuadorian Andes* (1988).

In the meantime Westerners' increasing awareness of the calamitous consequences of overproduction and undernutrition throughout the world food system stimulated a number of predominantly biological anthropologists to work within the confines of a new sub-field they termed 'nutritional anthropology'. Its development was further encouraged in the late-1970s and early-1980s by the United Nations University and UNICEF; both offered assistance to anthropologists who were concerned with nutritional issues in any part of the globe, whether industrialised or not. The biological anthropologists, Stanley Ulijaszek and Simon Strickland (1993: 1), have defined this new sub-field as 'the study of human diet and nutrition within a comparative and evolutionary perspective'. Typical work carried out by nutritional anthropologists involves the assessment and further development of programmes of nutrition and primary health care. Some focus on the interactions between genes, physiological processes, population characteristics and a host of nutrition-related diseases, while others concentrate on the interrelationships among community health programmes, dietary patterns and other facets of local cultures (Pelto *et al.* 1989). In 1980 the nutritional anthropologists Randy Kandel, Gretel Pelto and Norge Jerome somewhat brazenly declared that their sub-field had already yielded 'new insights into areas which could barely be foreseen five years ago. These include:

1. a new perspective on the cultural sensitivity of nutritional standards and the question of biological adaptation,
2. the role of maternal feeding practices in fostering differential nutritional status among children within a single socioeconomic community,
3. the role of social networks in changing dietary models,
4. the nutritional implications of the cognitive structure of meal planning,
5. the impact of dietary anomalies, such as chronic hypoglycemia, in influencing the culture focus of entire isolated ethnic groups,
6. the precise description of the behavioral consequences of differential nutritional status' (Kandel *et al.* 1980: 6).

Nine years later the Peltos and Ellen Messer felt able to proclaim that the patent value of the interdisciplinary methods employed by nutritional anthropologists had quickly been taken on board by nutritional epidemiologists and those who wished to carry out nutrition surveys (Pelto *et al.* 1989).

From the late-1980s, within social anthropology, a version of postmodernism enjoyed some popularity. Its main value was to make many anthropologists far more conscious of the inescapably literary nature of everything they wrote. However, this 'literary turn' within the subject failed to fulfil its revolutionary promise; to its critics, it only resulted in work even more rarified than before. What is perhaps surprising is that its predictable demise, which started in the mid-1990s, chimed with the belated re-emergence of a 'socially relevant' or 'public' anthropology. In Britain at least this shift is to an important extent a consequence of a shift in funding priorities by the major foundations and above all the research councils of their government. British academics, under pressure from their universities which are in turn being financially squeezed, strive increasingly to win research grants which will help balance their departmental budget. A likely way to secure funds is to investigate topics which fit the funders' agendas for research which they regard as socially relevant. In this context of an ever more hard-nosed pragmatism, an anthropology of food can assume a level of significance previously denied. This current rage for 'relevance' has helped to move, if not to push, the anthropology of food towards the centre-stage of the subject, and this time in a purposefully interdisciplinary guise.

A modern anthropology of food has a very broad remit. It may include human dietary needs and traditional dietaries, hedonic responses and hedonism, subsistence strategies and ideologies of food, famine and cultures of consumption, the aid industry and Western food disorders, agricultural organisation and McDonaldisation. If, as Ahmed and Shore (1995: 15) claim, contemporary anthropology is saddled with a problem of relevance, then anthropologists of food are particularly well-positioned to respond to that challenge. Two examples will suffice here. First, it is a commonly stated fear that the ever-increasing spread of American fast-food franchises will affect both culinary variety and nutritional adequacy throughout the world. Yet, as Watson (1997) and his contributors argue, in East Asia locals have managed to adapt these outlets to their own particular ends and so make them, in some sense, their own. Globalisation is vanquished, at least for the time being. (But see Messer's chapter, this volume, for criticisms of Watson's book). Second, Pottier (1999) contends that over the last decade anthropology has been at the forefront of debate about food and food policy, informing discussions about food security, injecting new life into debates on 'free market' policy and 'real' markets, and proffering novel insights into the nature of biodiversity. What is now needed is for anthropologists of food to exploit their expertise in order to extend and deepen their participation in relevant public debates (e.g. Messer and Shipton 2002).

## Why Bother with Interdisciplinarity?

It is important to emphasise at this point that anthropologists of food are not obliged to perform in an interdisciplinary manner. There is nothing necessary about the process. A good number of noteworthy studies in the anthropology of food have been carried out within the confines of a single discipline: the food-centred *Mythologiques* of Lévi-Strauss (1964, 1967, 1969) are the best example here. It is just that so many of the questions we pose are best answered by utilising the strengths of different disciplines. This is primarily because, for humans, food can be regarded as both 'nature' and 'culture'. The same cannot be said for any other animal. No other primate knows anything about culinary operations. The one possible exception is the macaque (*Macaca fuscata*) monkey of Japan which may dip its potatoes into saltwater before consumption. No primates other than humans know how to use fire for gastronomic ends; there are no chefs in nonhuman primate societies. Only we humans have complex ways of preparing foods, which we pass on to our children. Gorillas and chimpanzees have well-developed brains but they do not have recipes. The staff at London Zoo might stage a Chimps' Tea Party but what exactly the chimpanzees think they are doing during this performance is another matter (MacClancy 1993). Samuel Johnson made much the same point, much more pungently, over two hundred years ago:

I had found out a perfect definition of human nature as distinguished from the animal. An ancient philosopher said, Man was 'a two-legged animal without feathers', upon which his rival sage had a cock plucked bare, and set down in the school before all his disciples as a 'Philosophick Man'. Dr (Benjamin) Franklin said, Man was 'a tool-making animal', which is very well; for no animal but man makes a thing. But this applies to very few of the species. My definition of Man is a 'Cooking Animal'. The beasts have memory, judgement, and all the facilities and passions of our mind, in a certain degree; but no beast is a cook (from Boswell 1970: 179, fn.1).

For humans, food bridges many divides: it is both substance and symbol; it is life-sustaining in both biochemical and cognitive modes. Both physically and socially, we consume it and make it part of ourselves, only to expel it in another form. In other words, for all of us, food is both nutrition and a mode of thought. Lévi-Strauss said it better: 'Food is not only good to eat, but also good to think with'. By definition, nothing else in human life fits that double bill.

Within the anthropology of food, interdisciplinarity is neither obligatory nor new. In the 1930s Richards was already working in an interdisciplinary manner, as she had botanists, nutritionists and biochemists help her to identify and assess the nutritional values of foods.

There are almost as many ways of practising interdisciplinarity as there are practitioners of it. The specific mode of interdisciplinarity employed is decided anew with each particular project. Sharp-eyed readers of this book will notice that several contributors have their own particular conceptions of inter-, multi-, pluri- or cross-disciplinarity. The choice of term is somewhat arbitrary, as each contributor has the same ultimate goal: for each project embarked upon, the overall aim, if we are to answer the questions we pose, is to be inter-disciplinary in a rigorous fashion, not merely multidisciplinary in an un-integrated manner. When dealing with one particular problem within the anthropology of food, the goal is not just to 'stack' different approaches (e.g. nutritional, ethnobotanical, social anthropological) on top of one another, as though their simple contiguity would lend power to one's argument. For each problem tackled, what researchers have to demonstrate is how different approaches may be linked productively. They may well have to perceive links that no one has shown before. The links made may well be different when dealing with different problems. They cannot usually be prescribed, only teased out as the research progresses. But unless persuasive sets of links *are* made the result is merely an undisciplined multidisciplinarity, not a rigorous interdisciplinarity.

## Exemplars of Multidisciplinary Food Studies

One patent corollary to the above is that what anthropologists of food need is the intellectual boldness to be able to think beyond the conventional bound-aries of individual disciplines, and to combine approaches in a creative, con-structive manner. We shall give two examples.

The anthropologist, Sidney Mintz, in his magisterial study, *Sweetness and Power*, (1985), analysed the way sugar was converted from being a luxury condiment for the powerful to becoming the first proletarian staple of modern industrialised society. To carry out this work meant researching the evolution of sugar production in the Caribbean, the development of its consumption in Britain and the unfolding interaction between these two poles: an interaction which aided the creation and consolidation of a truly world capitalism. Rather than focus on just one small-scale face-to-face community — the sugar plantation where he had done his original fieldwork in the late 1940s — Mintz took a more global, evolutionary perspective. At the time, it was a pioneering move. Moreover, in the course of this prize-winning analysis, he drew in a consistently imaginative manner from the work of human biologists, nutritionists, social historians and social anthropologists. In doing so, and in doing it so successfully, Mintz helped to prefigure a modern anthropology.

Our second exemplar is by an even more inventive synthesiser. Jared Diamond's bestselling *Guns, Germs and Steel: a short history of everybody for the last 13,000 years* (1997) has made him one of the most well-known scientific popularisers of recent decades. As global in aim as the subtitle suggests, Diamond sets himself the big questions: why has so much of history taken the course it has? Why has it unfolded so differently on different continents? To answer these, he relies on work done by geneticists, molecular biologists, food biogeographers, ethnobiologists, epidemiologists, archaeologists, linguists and social anthropologists, among others. Most historians present history as the consequence of human decisions. What gives Diamond's work its edge is that he portrays history in broad terms, as a consequence of the interaction between humans and the different environments within which they live. Particular environments enable human groups to develop in certain ways: people in certain areas can grow certain kinds and combinations of crops; they can hunt certain animals and may be able to domesticate some of them; interaction with these animals may give them resistance to certain diseases; and all of these factors may have immediate and radical consequences for those peoples and the elaboration of their societies. It is as though his environmentalism gently mocked the pretensions of those historians who present humans as the independent makers of their own destiny.

Pedants might quibble that Diamond is not in fact an anthropologist of food. It is true that his academic position is not in anthropology; he is a professor of physiology at the University of California Medical School. But that fact serves us in making an important point. Because the anthropology of food is an almost open-ended interdisciplinary melange, it may well be the case that academics, from whatever particular university faculty, working within or very near this general area will conduct interdisciplinary investigations which, in terms of methods, overlap greatly with those associated with the anthropology of food. The point remains: we should not be concerned with the pettiness of academic turf wars, but aim to find revealing answers to the important questions we pose. In this context, exactly which disciplinary badge one wears is almost irrelevant. We have entitled this book *Researching Food Habits: methods and problems* and we flatter ourselves that its lessons may be of value to any student researching the human use of food.

## This Book

We wanted to include as broad a range of approaches as possible, in order to give students and new researchers an idea of just how diverse the anthropology of food is and how many different sets of methods anthropologists of food might employ. However, of necessity some perspectives are neglected. Although there is some grouping of the chapters, the editors do not perceive clear enough subdivisions to create named sections.

The first chapter is by one of the most senior and productive of anthropologists of food. For decades de Garine has worked in and led multidisciplinary teams investigating problems in the anthropology of food. He makes the excellent point that for biological scientists and social scientists to work alongside each other can be a very tricky business as they tend to have different expectations, different criteria of validity and significance, and different timetables. These difficulties are not a peculiarly European problem, as American anthropologists have confirmed experiencing similar difficulties, often compounded by the negative stereotypes each group of academics may hold of the others (Kandel *et al.* 1980). Nevertheless, de Garine has successfully led a team which has cooperated for many years, even in the field, across the biological/social science divide.

Szabó's chapter on ethnobotanical methods emphasises the central importance of taking local people seriously, of listening to what they have to say and writing it down on paper. All too often, up until very recently, botanists studying the regional flora of an area have not bothered to ask the locals how they classify and understand the plants in their surroundings. Yet, if the environment within which people live is a historical product of the sustained interaction between plants, animals, humans and their technology, then it is surely incumbent on ecologically oriented researchers to find out how locals perceive the world around them. The categories within which they think help form their thought, their thoughts inform their actions and their actions affect the environment. This chapter provides a practical guide on the collection and preservation of plant material in the field and its analysis in the laboratory, as well as tuition on how to gain as much information as possible from local informants on their naming and use of the plants.

Some of the more quantitatively inclined among social scientists like to criticise social anthropologists for their apparently vague, qualitative approach. Stung by these barbs, some social anthropologists brand their critics as naïve empiricists overkeen on arithmetical results and mathematical models. In this unnecessarily common exchange of verbal abuse, the protagonists lampoon each other as 'number-crunchers' ranked against the 'woolly-headed', supposedly more interested in impressions than precision. However, in the third chapter, Hubert boldly tries to steer a middle course by suggesting a method whereby the two research styles might be combined and their complementary strengths exploited. This clearly didactic chapter gives explicit advice on each step new researchers should take in carrying out such research. An appendix to the chapter provides a guide to topics that can usefully be raised in interviews about food and drink patterns in a household. Her approach shows the value of visiting households and the rooms where food is prepared and served, in order to observe food producers at their sites of production.

The central feature of any social approach is talk. Researchers and locals talk to one another. In that way researchers learn things that they did not know before, which they write down and can later analyse to produce findings and conclusions. If this approach is to work, there must be some trust, however minimal, between researchers and the people with whom they talk. In fact, social anthropology is the only discipline whose main research method is also its goal: to learn about social relationships ethnographers have first to create social relationships with the people they are studying. Medina's chapter focuses on this interaction between researchers and researched. He teases out part of the nature and some of the consequences of this complex, ever-dynamic form of relationship. The possible pitfalls of this kind of fieldwork may be great, but the rewards, when they are achieved, can be even greater.

In much social anthropology today, the topic of 'identity' looms large. What is not always mentioned by those happy to use the concept is that it brings with it a whole train of difficulties. MacClancy, in his contribution, strives to forewarn fledgling researchers of these danger points, and how best to avoid them. He then plots the various avenues that fresh fieldworkers might wish to pursue. He particularly dwells on frequently ignored, but very useful, sources of information, such as newspaper articles, novels and past and current cookbooks. Why such potentially fruitful sources of material have so often been passed over is a puzzle yet to be solved.

A big temptation for teachers of method is to present the course of fieldwork as virtually flawless and relatively untroubled. A prevailing orthodoxy among too many lecturers who teach anthropological research methods is that yes, one may have initial difficulties with the locals, and yes, certain rituals may be hidden from the researcher's view, but if the fieldworker stays long enough most of these difficulties should simply pass away. Teachers of this kind seem keener to sing the praises of fieldwork than to depict its dirty realism: gaps in the data gathered, worries about the status of some of their data, concerns about the questions left unasked and doubts about information partly remembered but not written down at the time, etc. Gerald and Valerie Mars's contribution is so valuable, because this – the dirty realism – is precisely the problem they dwell on. To our knowledge this is the first time the question has been so openly broached for publication. What they show, in two highly appropriate examples, is that we cannot always live up to the standards that we have been trained to set ourselves. There will always be some occasions when we have to gather what information we can – however impoverished it might appear – because the particular opportunity will not arise again. In these events we must do what we can, given that we can do no more; our results may still be of great value. To put that another way, our work may yet produce interesting and valuable results even though our final statements may not be as securely based as we should wish. This the Mars call 'the good enough principle'.

In the next chapter, Simmen, Pasquet and Hladik show how to assess (1) gustatory perception (taste on the tongue) by determining taste thresholds, and (2) hedonic reactions to tastes by using supra-threshold responses. They outline methods for use in the laboratory and those that can be taken into the field. This might at first seem a sudden switch from the social towards the strictly biological. Not so. As Hladik and Simmen (1996) pointed out with respect to humans and food, even aspects of human life thought to be purely biological cannot be neatly separated from culturally learned responses. They do not limit their instruction on methods to research on humans, but also include an explanation of methods for testing nonhuman primates. They suggest that those who wish to understand the basic qualities of the human tasting phenomenon can gain a useful, evolutionary perspective from the study of the reactions of nonhuman primates. In this chapter, the contributors argue that the taste system is a primary interface between an organism and its alimentary environment, and it is, therefore, an integral part of the physiological back-ground from which feeding behaviour and food habits have developed. Thus, investigating hedonic responses fosters understanding both of the original inter-face and of the contemporary ways in which cultural conditions interact with human physiology.

Macbeth and Mowatt's chapter follows straight on from this, as they look into the problems which arise when trying to research hedonic responses across different cultures. The topic of preferences that humans express about different food items is much broader than the physiological reactions on tongue and other neurological pathways, because of strong sociocultural influences. As they state, biochemical processes and social experiences are in-extricably linked. Furthermore, researchers who want to study food prefer-ences and aversions outside of their own society have to be very sensitive to potential cultural and linguistic differences, and for those, who in one study wish to *compare* the food preferences of people from different cultures, there is a diversity of complexities, some very subtle. Whereas statistically complex methods for reducing statements about food preferences to quantitative data have been used before, these methods had been designed for research within one society. The problem which Macbeth and Mowatt tackle is how to design a method appropriate for comparing food preferences across five sample popu-lations, each from a different European nation. Although they chose to use questionnaires, these were of a very special format, which owed much to careful prior fieldwork, interviewing and trials in each of the countries. Their method and their conclusions about that method are given in detail in this chapter, and they warn that not all the complexities are resolved by use of this kind of method; researchers should also spend time with the subjects being studied, discussing with them and observing their attitudes.

Ulijaszek makes a similar set of caveats in the next chapter, where he very skilfully plots the diverse pitfalls in studies of dietary intake. Indeed his depressing but illuminating contribution reads more like a sceptic's essay, or as an extended series of cautionary tales for those with more enthusiasm than patience. Ulijaszek's necessary message appears to be: fledgling researcher be aware!

More information on food intake studies follows in the chapter by Henry and Macbeth. After an overview of nutritionists' methods for studying food intake, they focus on the gathering of food intake frequency data. They then introduce in detail one low-budget, macrosurvey method for studying 7-day food intake frequency. As they point out, their inexpensive method does not aim to provide nutritional precision but an initial quantitative overview of foods eaten in the course of one week. They suggest that this sort of quick survey can be a very useful supplement to ethnographic work. For, as they bluntly state, 'the researcher cannot be in every kitchen and dining room of a study population all the time'. The method is useful when precision about nutrients, weights and quantities is less important than an overall, quantified description of food intake either in a larger population sample or for the comparison of more than one population.

One significant aspect of human nutritional status is energy balance. This is the difference between energy intake and energy expenditure. Since Henry and Macbeth's chapter included mention of energy intake, calculated from food intake, Pasquet's chapter is the perfect complement, because he discusses methods for measuring energy expenditure. Pasquet provides detailed information on the measuring of energy expenditure, a methodology which has developed greatly within biological anthropology. The idea of energy balance within a whole community has also been used by human ecologists, when they study the patterns of energy intake and expenditure involved in that population's consumption of food and methods of production and distribution, in their particular environment.

The contributions in the next two chapters take on a more historical twist. Their authors emphasise the need for diverse research methods and co-operation between specialists from different disciplines. González, a social anthropologist, and Mataix, a nutritionist, describe their very sensitive and imaginative way of obtaining quantitative data about a particular local diet in the first half of the twentieth century. They approach the question from three different angles, linking oral interview data from elderly women with information from equally elderly trades people, who were at the time concerned with purveying the basic foodstuffs, and finally converting these data, measured in spoonfuls, cupfuls, handfuls, etc., to modern measurements for comparison with nutrient tables. They detail, with exemplary utility, the indispensable safeguards to be taken when interviewing aged people about circumstances in their youth or even in their adolescence. The next contributor, Pollock, tackles a related set of problems in reconstructing a local diet by exploiting every source possible: written accounts of the society's past, plant and food inventories, historical settings, earlier ethnography, personal knowledge of community members and suggestive cross-cultural comparisons. Exemplifying the interdisciplinary aim of this book, she shows how her work on one particular project dovetailed with that of the health physicists involved, so that together they produced a broader understanding than either specialism alone could have provided.

This volume ends, appropriately, by ceding the final chapter to a distinguished North American colleague, Ellen Messer, whose research and writings on the anthropology of food have been a beacon to us all. She opens her contribution with a brief but magisterial critique of certain ethnographic styles in contemporary studies of the anthropology of food. Then her main example, from fieldwork in Mexico, demonstrates 'ways to collect dietary information so that it can provide both cultural and biological insights, even without additional anthropometrical or laboratory studies'. Her constructively critical discussion shows the sorts of information and analysis needed for this kind of work.

## A Time for Conclusion?

It was Messer (1984) who, in a major review, observed that collaborative efforts between anthropologists, psychologists and biologists seemed to be increasing. She went on to call for more interdisciplinary work within the general field of the anthropology of food. Late in the next decade Pottier noted that anthropological 'interest in food, agriculture, food security and health is peaking'. He hoped anthropology would become 'fit to provide guidance in a fast-changing world' (Pottier 1999: 9). What they, among many others, wished to see was more work done in the area and for more of this work to be policy-relevant.

We agree. That is why we edited this book, which we see as a chest of intellectual tools for would-be researchers to pick up and use and develop. Interest in the topic continues to rise. The challenge is there; the time is now. This is no place for a conclusion.

## Acknowledgements

We wish to thank Catherine Hill for comments on an earlier draft.

# References

Ahmed, A.S. and Shore, C.N. (1995) Is Anthropology Relevant to the Contemporary World? In Ahmed, A. and Shore, C. (eds) *The Future of Anthropology: Its Relevance to the Contemporary World*, Athlone, London, 12–45.

Boswell, J. (1970) *Journal of a Tour to the Hebrides with Samuel Johnson, L.L.D.*, (edition edited by R.W.Chapman), Oxford University Press, Oxford.

Diamond, J. (1997) *Guns, Germs and Steel: A short history of everybody for the last 13,000 years*, Chatto and Windus, London.

Douglas, M. (1966) *Purity and Danger*, Routledge and Kegan Paul, London.

Firth, R. (1934) The sociological study of native diet, *Africa*, 7(4): 74–78.

Fortes, M. and Fortes, S.L. (1936) Food in the domestic economy of the Tallensi, *Africa*, 9: 237–76.

Freedman, R. L. (1977) Nutritional Anthropology: An Overview. In Fitzgerald, T.K. (ed.) *Nutrition and Anthropology in Action*, van Gorcum, Assen/Amsterdam, 1–23.

Guthe, C. E. and Mead, M. (1945) Manual for the Study of Food Habits, *Bulletin of the National Research Council*, National Academy of Sciences, Washington, D.C. No. 111.

Harris, M. (1966) The Cultural Ecology of India's Sacred Cattle, *Current Anthropology*, 7: 51–66.

Harris, M. (1979) *Cultural Materialism: The Struggle for a Science of Culture*, Random House, New York.

Harris, M. (1987) *The Sacred Cow and the Abominable Pig: Riddles of food and culture*, Simon Schuster, New York. [Originally published in 1985 as *Good to Eat*].

Harris, M. and Ross, E.B. (eds) (1987) *Food and Evolution: Toward a theory of human food habits*, Temple University Press, Philadelphia.

Hladik, C.M. and Simmen, B. (1996) Taste perception and feeding behavior in nonhuman primates and human populations, *Evolutionary Anthropology*, 5: 58–71.

Kandel, R., Jerome, N., and Pelto, G. (1980) Introduction. In Jerome, N., Kandel, R. and Pelto, G. (eds) *Nutritional Anthropology: Contemporary approaches to diet and culture*, Redgrave, New York, 1–11.

Lévi-Strauss, C. (1964) *Mythologiques, volume 1, Le cru et el cuit*, Plon, Paris.

Lévi-Strauss, C. (1967) *Mythologiques, volume 2, Du miel aux cendres*, Plon, Paris.

Lévi-Strauss, C. (1969) *Mythologiques, volume 3, L'origine des manières de table*, Plon, Paris.

MacClancy, J. (1986) Unconventional character and disciplinary convention: John Layard, Jungian and Anthropologist. In Stocking, G. (ed.) *Malinowski, Rivers, Benedict and Others: Essays on culture and personality, History of Anthropology*, volume 4, University of Wisconsin Press, Madison, 50–71.

MacClancy, J. (1993) *Consuming Culture*, Henry Holt, New York.

MacClancy, J. (1995) Brief Encounter: the meeting, in Mass-Observation, of British surrealism and popular anthropology, *Journal of the Royal Anthropological Institute* (n.s.), 1(3): 495–512.

MacClancy, J. (1996) Popularizing Anthropology. In MacClancy, J. and McDonaugh, C. (eds) *Popularizing Anthropology*, Routledge, London, 1–57.

Mead, M. (1943a) Dietary patterns and food habits, *Journal of the American Dietetic Association*, 19: 1–5.

Mead, M. (1943b) The factor of food habits, *Annals of the American Academy of Political Science*, 225: 136–141.

Messer, E. (1984) Anthropological Perspectives on Diet, *Annual Review of Anthropology*, 13: 205–49.

Messer, E. and Shipton, P. (2002) Hunger in Africa: Untangling its Human Roots. In MacClancy, J.V. (ed.) *Exotic No More: Anthropology on the front lines,* University of Chicago Press, Chicago, 227–250.

Mintz, S. (1985) *Sweetness and Power,* Viking Penguin, New York.

Pelto, G.H., Pelto, P.J. and Messer, E. (eds) (1989) *Research methods in nutritional anthropology,* United Nations University Publications, Tokyo (Also available in e-version at http://www.unu.edu/unupress/unupbooks/80632e/80632E00.htm).

Pottier, J. (1999) *Anthropology of Food: The social dynamics of food security,* Polity, Cambridge.

Richards, A. (1932) *Hunger and Work in a Savage Tribe: A functional study of nutrition among the southern Bantu,* Routledge, London.

Richards, A. (1939) *Land, Labour and Diet in Northern Rhodesia: An economic study of the Bemba tribe*, Oxford University Press, Oxford.

Service, E. (1962) *Primitive Social Organization*, Random House, New York.

Steward, J. (1955), *Theory of Culture Change*, University of Illinois Press, Urbana.

Stocking, G.W., Jr. (1988) Bones, Bodies, and Behaviour. In Stocking, G.W., Jr (ed.) *Bones, Bodies, and Behaviour: Essays in biological anthropology; History of Anthropology,* volume 4, University of Wisconsin Press, Madison, 3–17.

Stocking, G.W., Jr. (2001) *Delimiting Anthropology: Occasional essays and reflections,* University of Wisconsin Press, Madison.

Ulijaszek, S. and Strickland, S. (1993) *Nutritional Anthropology: Prospects and perspectives*, Smith-Gordon, Nishimura.

Watson, J. (ed.) (1997) *Golden Arches East: McDonalds in East Asia,* Stanford University Press, Palo Alto.

Weismantel, M. (1988) *Food, Gender and Poverty in the Ecuadorian Andes,* University of Pennsylvania Press, Philadelphia.

# 1. ANTHROPOLOGY OF FOOD AND PLURIDISCIPLINARITY

*Igor de Garine*

## Biology and Culture

Humans consume food to fulfil a primary biological need, but they are not only directed by this biological need. Omnivorous creatures, they can satisfy their nutritional needs by using a very broad range of foods. They can have a largely vegetarian diet, like the inland populations of New Guinea (Oomen and Corden 1970), or they may consume mostly animal foods, as among the Inuit of the Arctic (Draper 1977), in order to reach an acceptable, if not necessarily optimal, diet according to contemporary nutritional standards as defined by Western scientists. Some groups appear to be more successful than others in their nutrition.

Humans are social animals, endowed with symbolic thinking, who in their societies elaborate a culture, a dynamic corpus of knowledge and material arte-facts, which is transmitted from generation to generation. Their attitudes and behaviour in relation to food are largely a product of a learning process in the framework of their own society and culture. Guthe and Mead (1945: 13) referred to this aspect when they defined food habits as ' ...the way in which individuals or groups of individuals, in response to social and cultural processes select, consume and utilise portions of the available food supply'. The last part of this quotation suggests that, contrary to what many might think, the ultimate aim of human diets is *not* automatically to achieve the best possible inclusive biological fitness through the use of all of the food resources avail-able.

Each society makes its choices among the potential food items according to a broad range of original factors. Within these choices each individual oper-ates their own selection according to personal criteria. It is necessary to take into account that, besides biological and sociocultural aspects, there is a psy-chological dimension to feeding behaviour: the influence of early and specific life experiences of each individual. Since this book is concerned with humans as social animals, rather than as individuals, I shall not deal with this aspect here.

## Society, Culture and Food Systems

In each society and in each subgroup it is usually more or less possible to distinguish an established consensus (which may vary over time) about what is normal, beneficial or negative in terms of food. Attempts by anthropologists to define this cultural common denominator normally necessitate a pluridisciplinary approach. It is necessary to learn who eats what, how much, when, where, with whom and, especially, why, and with what biological and psychological results. In general terms, the anthropology of food and nutrition implies a holistic approach to the biological, cultural and psychological factors concerning food behaviour and resulting in the nutritional and health status of a human group. Material artefacts as well as non-material systems of beliefs are involved.

## Food Themes among Anthropologists

For a long time social anthropologists did not show much interest in the field of food, with the result that most anthropological books contain only a little scattered information and no systematic studies of this subject. In the 1930s, Firth (1934) and Malinowski (1935) devoted more interest to this domain. The latter stimulated Audrey Richards to study from a functionalist perspective the cultural and social function of the food-getting process among the Bemba of Northern Rhodesia (now Zambia). Her first book, *Hunger and Work in a Savage Tribe* (Richards 1932) was followed by *Land, Labour and Diet in Northern Rhodesia* (Richards 1939), which was more oriented towards applied problems. Another approach developed in the United States under Second World War pressures, when Guthe and Mead created, in 1941, the Committee for the Study of Food Habits. This was intended to help countries where people were starving and also to allow allied military personnel to subsist abroad. They issued the first *Manual for the Study of Food Habits* in 1945 (Guthe and Mead 1945).

At much the same time, neo-Freudian anthropologists based in America, who formed part of the 'culture and personality school' attempted to show the importance of food and the frustration it, along with sex, may exert on the type of personality thought to be characteristic of various cultures (e.g. Kardiner 1939, Kardiner *et al.* 1945).

The concern of functionalist anthropologists to take into account ecology and material aspects of culture led to closer study of the food quest. Researchers from various schools of thought, such as cultural ecology (Kroeber

1939, Steward 1959) and utilitarianism (White 1949) looked at subsistence activities as a central and dynamic aspect of culture. Cultural materialists, such as Marvin Harris, whose work (e.g. 1978) has proved extremely popular, further developed this line of investigation. This generation of anthropologists was followed by a contingent of human ecologists concerned with the study of energy flow, of which food is a basic component (see Henry and Macbeth this volume, Pasquet this volume). These human ecologists focused mostly on hunter-gatherers (Lee and De Vore 1968, Rappaport 1968, Vayda 1969, Sahlins 1972, Thomas *et al.* 1979, Winterhalder 1993). The great concern shown by so many these days in environmental issues has contributed to maintaining an interest which is global in scope.

Structural anthropologists, led by Lévi-Strauss (1965), adopted a totally different viewpoint: they identified food as a major topic of investigation, which expressed unconsciously the deep structural features of society. Structuralists, however, remained within the intellectual domain of symbolism and did not bother much to look at 'objective' aspects of food consumption. A few human ecologists, working individually, attempted to gain a systematic outlook on the nutrition of the populations they studied, and gathered some quantitative data. For instance, Rappaport (1968), working among the Tsembaga of New Guinea, obtained quantitative food consumption data for sixteen persons over a period of 246 days, while Lee (1979) weighed and measured a sample of 215 !Kung San of the Kalahari during both the season of plenty (July) and that of scarcity (October). Rappaport's study was a one-man show, whereas, for some of the time, Lee's involved colleagues who were biologists. Both emphasised the need for quantitative data on food consumption and Lee suggested that the easiest way was 'to weigh the people periodically rather than to struggle laboriously to monitor their food intake' (Lee 1979: 282). Many biologists still agree with this view. Others disagree.

Rappaport was severely criticised by McArthur (1977) on the grounds that food consumption surveys are too laborious to be carried out by isolated researchers and need to be undertaken by professional nutritionists. To date, Pagézy (1988) may be one of the only individual fieldworkers providing acceptable quantitative data on diet together with reliable observations of an ethnological and biological anthropological nature.

## Need for Collaboration

Collaboration between nutritional and cultural anthropologists may be the answer to these criticisms. This is not easy to manage. For a long time the collaborative work achieved by Richards and Widdowson (1936) among the Bemba remained unparalleled.

The reasons for this are not only technical. Margaret Mead, referring to the creation of the Committee for the Study of Food Habits during the Second World War, writes: 'In this time of national emergency there was a greater willingness than is usually the case to extend to the newer behavioral sciences the kind of recognition given to older disciplines such as nutrition, biochemistry and medicine' (Mead 1964: 2). She was indicating a problem which has not totally disappeared today, the lack of mutual recognition between biologists and social scientists. Biologists deal with seemingly objective material data, some of which is easily measurable, but they are not usually trained to establish human contacts. Social anthropologists tend to investigate verbal, non-material and symbolic factors which are difficult to quantify. 'Hard' scientists are dubious about the scientific validity of the work of 'soft' social scientists, who in turn do not consider their colleagues to be very subtle and object to the intrusiveness of their techniques upon the populations under study.

I would like to argue that if we are to attain any progress in the study of human nutrition, a holistic approach is needed when looking at the nutritional adaptability of human beings. In his work on the !Kung San in 1979, Lee collaborated with biological anthropologists (Truswell and Hansen 1976). Later, to quote the example I know best, in France, Koppert (a nutritionist) teamed up with de Garine, which resulted in a series of integrated papers, (see for instance, Garine and Koppert 1988, 1990, 1991). The pluridisciplinary team on the Anthropology of Food of the French National Scientific Research Centre (CNRS) was created by mutual cooperation of its team members, which included biological anthropologists (Froment 1996), nutritionists (Koppert 1996) and cultural anthropologists. They managed to collaborate for over fifteen years, often working together in difficult environments on fourteen different Cameroonian tribes – and these researchers still talk to each other!

## The Cultural Anthropological Focus

What needs to be observed to gain an understanding of the food quest? Obviously, whatever appears to be directly connected to food, such as food consumption. More remote factors may also impinge upon feeding behaviour, for instance the family budget, priorities in terms of expenses, etc. One example will suffice. The Masa of Northern Cameroon are said to be 'cattle crazy' since cattle are the basis of bridewealth and prestige. As a consequence they may give priority to feeding their calves rather than to giving the milk to their own children. Most of their spare money goes towards buying cattle rather than to obtaining food stores for the hunger period which will inevitably occur. This food insecurity may well be the reason why the Masa utilise unsieved flour containing indigestible phytates, which rapidly produces a feeling of satiation.

The data to be obtained in research depend, of course, on the purpose of the study. One does not scrutinise the same aspects if one is looking for causes of malnutrition rather than for causes of anxiety in relation to food pollution or for preferences in relation to a given kind of foodstuff. It is, nevertheless, wise to keep a broad outlook upon various aspects of the culture studied while

*Figure 1.1*   Igor de Garine interviewing respondents in the field

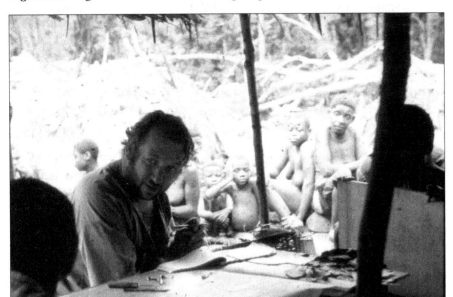

focusing on the pertinent aspects. As Mauss pointed out ([1923] 1950), there are 'total social phenomena' which may set in motion or refer to any aspect of the material and non-material culture. This is the case when food is fundamental to a social event. So, while food choices may not necessarily reach or aim at optimal nutritional results, they may still fulfil important, non-material, cultural goals.

## A Tentative Checklist

In view of the above, a tentative check list can be provided for new researchers of useful aspects to consider when studying the anthropology of food:

   I.     *General aspects* – environment; habitat; seasonal variations; demography.

   II.    *Quantitative nutritional aspects* – food consumption studies, at representative periods of the annual cycle, involving various categories and ages of individuals and including anthropometry; the analysis of relevant biochemical samples (from blood, urine, stools, etc.) and energy expenditure measures with time budgets. All the above should be obtained for the same periods over the year.

   III.   *Social anthropology of food* – the data should be obtained by direct observation, interviews and questionnaires. Two perspectives on each phenomenon should be taken into account – an outsider's perspective ('etic') and the way that the phenomenon is perceived by the population under consideration ('emic'). Social and cultural anthropologists should obtain information on material and non-material culture, for example:

a) Material culture: artefacts and techniques in relation to predation, production, and preservation; storage of food products; food technology; cooking and food (including liquids) consumption; and also family budgets with special reference to food and drink.

b) Non-material culture: for example, local cultural knowledge about local animals (ethnozoology) and about local plants (ethnobotany) (see Szabó, this volume); social and religious organisation in relation to food production and consumption; social and religious rituals involving food (offerings); prestige in relation to food (food as a link, food as a marker, food and body shape); traditional knowledge in relation to nutrition and health (ethnomedicine); opinions and attitudes (preferences and rejections in relation to food); analysis of food themes in the oral literature (myths, legends, tales, sayings, songs, rhymes) and in dreams.

IV. *Psychosocial aspects related to food* – the learning process (through family, peers or the media, etc.); psychological rewards and frustrations related to food; stress; food anxiety in terms of psychopathological aspects related to food (bulimia, anorexia). Health safety has become an important aspect in contemporary behaviour towards food. In a society of plenty, where food selection is mostly a matter of individual choice, these aspects are of increasing importance.

## Need for Quantification

As far as the advancement of scientific knowledge and basic research is concerned, quantification is needed, burdensome and costly endeavour though it may be, if biological and social human scientists are to engage in productive dialogue. Such research should not rely on 'quick and dirty' techniques (see Cameron and Van Staveren 1988). From the scientific point of view, it would be a great pity to miss a priviledged research opportunity in which nutrition, a phenomenon influenced by non-material aspects of culture (such as beliefs or stress caused by failure to reach specific cultural objectives), may have a direct impact on human biology. The biological factors of interest might range from the nutritional status of a whole population to the enzyme excretion of some individuals.

So, what is desirable is a multidisciplinary approach. This means, of course, that a pluridisciplinary study of food and nutrition must be organised according to the objectives of that study and, in the case of fundamental research, the hypotheses to be tested. There is no compulsive need, for example, to go through a painstaking quantitative study of food consumption and anthropometric measurements if the purpose is only to determine the preferences of a human group towards a given type of food.

## Motives Underlying Pluridisciplinary Studies

Pluridisciplinary studies on food and nutrition are, in many cases, motivated by practical concerns. The pioneer work of Richards and Widdowson (1936), as well as that of Firth (1934), reflected the concern of the colonial powers to maintaining, in a changing world, the local populations in an acceptable state of health and nutrition, in order that they could work and enjoy sufficient well-being. I already mentioned the influence of war on the development of research in the United States into food habits. At the end of the Second World War, generous attention was given to providing appropriate food to all human groups in the world in order to maintain an acceptable level of health. International agencies such as the World Health Organisation (WHO) and the Food and Agriculture Organisation (FAO) were created. Nutritional education programmes flourished as well as those for applied nutrition. In both cases it was necessary to look at the attitudes of the people towards foodstuffs, as well as at their nutritional status. The primary focus was on the nutritionally vulnerable groups such as children and pregnant women. Applied nutrition programmes consisted specifically of determining the nutritional needs of populations and the level of malnutrition. The aim of these programmes was to enable the people to reach a better diet by getting them to produce the needed commodities themselves and then to use them properly. Today, dietetic considerations are behind most of the pluridisciplinary projects. Some of these are concerned with the health of the general public; others are aimed at specific groups such as school children, soldiers, prisoners, hospitalised patients or particular individuals such as sportsmen or cosmonauts. More theoretical concerns, such as those of environmentalist groups, are also common today; for example, the search for 'natural' foods or psychological well-being through appropriate nourishment. As another example, it would be interesting to review the 'French Paradox' closely (see Glossary), in order to establish if there are any emotional, psychological factors involved besides the biochemical ones and if the general lifestyle is not concerned as well as the diet (Bourre 1990, Garine 1998).

## The Contemporary Vogue

Nowadays the anthropology of food is a fashionable topic and it has become customary to include a social scientist in biological field studies related to diet. A large amount of literature has been produced, among which a number of general books can be mentioned. For instance, there are Burgess and Dean (1962), Mead (1964), Yudkin and McKenzie (1964), Walcher *et al.* (1976), Fitzgerald (1977), Yudkin (1978), Farb and Armelagos (1980), Jerome, Kandel and Pelto (1980), Goody (1982), Harris and Ross (1987), Pelto *et al.* (1989), Geissler and Oddy (1993), MacClancy (1993), Den Hartog *et al.* (1995), Bataille-Benguigui and Cousin (1996), Lupton (1996), Counihan and van Esterik (1997), Guerci (1999), Museo Nacional de Antropología, España (1999) and Poulain (2002).

Books on historical aspects should also be mentioned. Among a very large number of titles, one could cite Burnett (1966), Chang (1977), Mennell (1985) and Flandrin and Montanari (1996).

Some bibliographies might also be noted, such as Wilson (1979) and Freedman (1981, 1983). A number of works deal with specific issues such as food taboos (Simoons 1994), disease (Harrison and Waterlow 1990), seasonality (Chambers *et al.* 1981, Garine and Harrison 1988), obesity (Garine and Pollock 1995), feasting (Douglas 1984), hunger (Bohle *et al.* 1991, 1993), status (Wiessner and Schiefenhövel 1995), food preferences (Macbeth 1997) and drinking (Garine and Garine 2001).

Publications bearing on specific areas of the world are many, but the following should also be mentioned; on Melanesia (Bayliss-Smith and Feachem 1977, Obrist Van Eewijk 1992), on Africa (Hladik *et al.* 1990, Froment *et al.* 1996), on China (Simoons 1991), on tropical forests (Hladik *et al.* 1993).

## Operational Aspects

The study of cultural aspects of food consumption is not just intrinsically interesting; it also provides important perspectives for biological studies. This cultural study may at the same time enable the realistic development of action programmes to improve the health of various groups within a population. It may also help to increase the sale of any type of commodity, foodstuff or trademark, where, for better or for worse, marketing has become a strong incentive for undertaking cultural studies on food choice and one of the main sources of financial support.

To be successful, any multidisciplinary study of food should be carefully planned ahead of time and be allowed a sufficient duration in order to achieve appropriate results in each of the fields considered. Although saving money on scientific research has become an all too common contemporary concern, to retain satisfactory scientific validity no study should be too superficial and simply provide data for computers.

In general, obtaining cross-disciplinary data in the field of human sciences takes longer than collecting information from only one perspective. In particular, work in a foreign culture implies an acceptable knowledge of the local language in order to communicate. It necessitates a thorough acquaintance with the people in order to establish sufficiently close bonds to avoid mistrust and misinformation. A practical solution is to develop a pluridisciplinary study on food where a cultural anthropological study has already been conducted and, if possible, to enlist the help of the cultural anthropologist concerned. If no ethnographic data are available and if the financial means allow, a useful protocol is for a cultural anthropologist to carry out research focusing on food aspects in the first year covering the full year cycle, and for the quantitative biological studies to take place during the second year.

As an example, the Anthropology of Food team of the French National Centre for Scientific Research (CNRS) (Garine and Koppert 1988, 1990, 1991, Hladik *et al.* 1990, 1993 and Froment *et al.* 1996) was able to carry out simultaneously a cultural anthropological investigation, a quantitative food consumption study encompassing the representative periods of the year in terms of food consumption, and a biological anthropological survey of nutrition, in several traditional populations. Luckily, the biological and cultural anthropologists did not tread on each other's toes during the field studies because of sufficient mutual respect, enough knowledge of each other's discipline, and sufficient size of the populations studied. Difficulties may arise during the processing of data and publication of results. Social scientists tend to take a longer time to process their data than biologists. The latter, in order to comply with the publishing style of their specialities, are eager to publish their results very rapidly before others publish similar results.

Producing an integrated work on the food system of a given population has been done by a number of pluridisciplinarily minded individual researchers, as we have mentioned above. What is more, different members of a pluridisciplinary team working on the same population or the same type of food problem are able to produce complementary papers appropriate for the journals of their own discipline. But, publishing a pluridisciplinary, integrated book on the anthropology of the food of a specific population, taking into account equally the biological and the cultural aspects of food and nutrition, has still to be achieved.

A last, essential aspect must be mentioned, and this involves a moral issue. It should be remembered that studying the feeding behaviour of a population represents an intrusion into the daily life and the privacy of its members, especially in periods of dearth. Taking into account the amount of nuisance which might be considered tolerable by the population and the extent to which that population will cooperate is an essential aspect of any study on food and nutrition, especially if it involves several field workers. This has been carried out, for instance, by the Anthropology of Food team of the CNRS (*op. cit.* above) in various Cameroonian ecosystems. Without the cooperation and understanding of the people we wish to study nothing can be done. We are, in the end, totally indebted to the people we work with.

# References

Bataille-Benguigui, A.C. and Cousin, F. (eds) (1996) *Cuisines, Reflets des Sociétés,* Editions Sépia, Musée de l'Homme, Paris: 9–28.

Bayliss-Smith, T. and Feachem, R. (eds) (1977) *Subsistence and Survival: Rural ecology in the Pacific,* Academic Press, London.

Bohle, H.B., Cannon, T., Hugo, G. and Ibrahim, F.N. (eds)(1991) Famine and food security in Africa and Asia : indigenous response and external intervention to avoid hunger, *Bayreuther Geowissenschaftliche Arbeiten,* 15, University of Bayreuth: 83–99.

Bohle, H.-G., Downing, T.E., Field, J.O. and Ibrahim, F.N. (eds)(1993) *Coping with Vulnerability and Criticality: case studies on food-insecure groups and regions,* Beitenbach Verlag, Saarbrücken: 339–359.

Bourre, J.D. (1990) *La Diététique du Cerveau: de l'Intelligence et du Plaisir,* Editions Odile Jacob, Paris.

Burgess, A. and Dean, R.F.A. (eds) (1962) *Malnutrition and Food Habits,* Tavistock, London.

Burnett, J. (1966) *Plenty and Want: a social history of diet in England from 1815 to the present day,* Pelican Books, Harmondsworth.

Cameron, M.E. and Van Staveren, W.A. (1988) *Manual on Methodology for Food Consumption Studies,* Oxford University Press, Oxford.

Chambers, R., Longhurst, R. and Pacey, A. (1981) *Seasonal Dimensions to Rural Poverty,* Francis Pinter, New York.

Chang, K.C. (ed.) (1977) *Food in Chinese culture – anthropological and historical perspectives,* Yale University Press, New Haven.

Counihan, C. and Van Esterik, R. (1997) *Food and Culture: a reader,* Routledge, London.

Den Hartog, A.P., Van Staveren, W.A. and Brouwer, I.D. (1995) *Manual for Social Surveys on Food Habits and Consumption in Developing Countries,* Margraf Verlag, Weikersheim, Germany.

Douglas, M. (ed.) (1984) *Food in the Social Order: studies of food and festivities in three American communities,* Sage Foundation, New York.

Draper, H. (1977) The aboriginal Eskimo diet in modern perspective, *American Anthropologist,* 79: 309–316.

Farb, P. and Armelagos, G. (1980) *Consuming Passions: the anthropology of eating,* Houghton Mifflin, Boston.

Firth, R. (1934) The sociological study of native diet, *Africa,* 7: 401–414.

Fitzgerald, T.K. (ed.) (1977) *Nutrition and Anthropology in Action,* Van Gocum, Assen, Amsterdam.

Flandrin, J.L and Montanari, M. (eds) (1996) *Histoire de l'Alimentation,* Fayard, Paris.

Freedman, R.L. (1981) *Human Food Uses: a cross cultural comprehensive annotated bibliography,* Greenwood Press, Westport, Connecticut.

Freedman, R.L. (1983) *Human Food Uses: a cross cultural comprehensive annotated bibliography (Supplement),* Greenwood Press, Westport, Connecticut.

Froment, A. (1996) Anthropologie alimentaire et biologie humaine. In Froment, A., Garine, I. de, Binam Bikoi, Ch., and Loung, J. F.(eds) *Bien Manger et Bien Vivre : Anthropologie alimentaire et développement en Afrique intertropicale: du biologique au social,* L'Harmattan, Office de la Recherche Scientifique et Technique, Outre-Mer, Paris: 35–48.

Froment, A., Garine, I. de, Binam Bikoi, Ch., and Loung, J.F. (eds) (1996) *Bien Manger et Bien Vivre. Anthropologie alimentaire et développement en Afrique intertropicale: du biologique au social,* L'Harmattan, Office de la Recherche Scientifique et Technique Outre-Mer, Paris.

Garine, I. de (1998) Views about food and culture in our contemporary world. In Cresta, M. and Teti, V. (eds) *The Road of Food Habits in the Mediterranean Area,* Rivista di Antropologia Supplement, 76, Publicazione dell'Istituto Italiano di Antropologia, Rome: 255–70.

Garine, I. de and Garine V. de, (eds) (2001) *Drinking: Anthropological Approaches,* Berghahn Books, Oxford.

Garine, I. de and Harrison, G.A. (eds) (1988) *Coping with Uncertainty in Food Supply,* Clarendon Press, Oxford.

Garine, I. de and Koppert, G.J.A. (1988) Coping with Seasonal Fluctuations in Food Supply among Savanna Populations: The Massa and Mussey of Chad and Cameroon. In Garine, I. de and Harrison, G.A. (eds) *Coping with Uncertainty in Food Supply,* Clarendon Press, Oxford: 210–260.

Garine, I. de and Koppert, G. (1990) Social Adaptation to Season and Uncertainty in Food Supply. In Harrison, G.A. and Waterlow, J.C. (eds) *Diet and Disease in Traditional and Developing Countries,* Cambridge University Press, Cambridge: 240–289.

Garine, I. de and Koppert, G.J.A. (1991) Guru – Fattening Sessions among the Massa, *Ecology of Food and Nutrition,* 25(1): 1–28.

Garine, I. de and Pollock, N.J. (eds) (1995) *Social Aspects of Fatness and Obesity,* Gordon and Breach, Amsterdam.

Geissler, C. and Oddy, D.J. (1993) *Diet and Economic Change, Past and Present,* Pinter, London.

Goody, J. (1982) *Cooking, Cuisine and Class: A study in comparative sociology,* Cambridge University Press, Cambridge.

Guerci, A. (ed.) (1999) *Il Cibo Culturale: dal cibo alla cultura, dalla cultura al cibo/Cultural Food: from food to culture, from culture to food,* Erga Edizioni, Genoa.

Guthe, C.E. and Mead, M. (1945) Manual for the Study of Food Habits, *Bulletin of National Research Council,* National Academy of Sciences, n° 111.

Harris, M. (1978) *Cannibals and Kings: the origins of culture,* Vintage Books, Random House, New York.

Harris, M. and Ross, E.B. (1987) *Food and Evolution : Towards a theory of human food habits,* Temple University Press, Philadelphia.

Harrison, G.A. and Waterlow, J.C. (eds) (1990) *Diet and Disease in Traditional Developing Societies,* Cambridge University Press, Cambridge.

Hladik, C.M., Bahuchet, S. and Garine, I. de (eds) (1990) *Food and Nutrition in the African Rain Forest,* Unesco/MAB, Paris.

Hladik, C.M., Pagézy, H., Linares, O.F., Hladik, A., Semple, A. and Hadley, M. (eds) (1993) *Tropical Forests, People and Food: biocultural interactions and applications to development,* Unesco/MAB, Paris.

Jerome, N.W., Kandel, R.F. and Pelto, G. (1980) *Nutritional Anthropology,* Redgrave, New York.

Kardiner A. (1939) *The Individual and his Society: the psychodynamics of primitive social organization*, Columbia University Press, New York.

Kardiner, A., Linton, R., Du Bois, C. and West, J. (1945) *The Psychological Frontiers of Society*, Columbia University Press, New York.

Koppert, G. (1996) Méthodologie de l'Enquête alimentaire. In Froment, A., Garine, I. de, Binam Bikoi, Ch. and Loung, J.F. (eds). *Bien Manger et Bien Vivre: anthropologie alimentaire et développement en Afrique intertropicale: du biologique au social*. L'Harmattan, Office de la Recherche Scientifique et Technique Outre-Mer, Paris: 89–98.

Kroeber A.L. (1939) *Cultural and Natural Areas of Native North America*, University of California Press, Berkeley.

Lee, R.B. (1979) *The !Kung San: Men, women and work in a foraging society*, Cambridge University Press, Cambridge.

Lee, R.B. and De Vore, I. (eds) (1968) *Man the Hunter*, Aldine, Chicago.

Levi-Strauss, C. (1965) Le triangle culinaire, *L'Arc*, 26: 19–29.

Lupton, D. (1996) *Food, the Body and the Self*, Sage, London.

Macbeth, H.M. (ed.) (1997) *Food Preferences and Taste: continuity and change*, Berghahn Books, Oxford.

MacClancy, J. (1993) *Consuming Culture*, Henry Holt, New York.

Malinowski, B. (1935) *Coral Gardens and their Magic: a study of the method of tilling the soil and of agricultural rites in the Trobriand Islands*, Allen and Unwin, London.

Mauss, M. (1923) Essai sur le don – forme et raison de l'échange dans les sociétés archaïques, *Année sociologique* 1923–1924, 2(1) [ 2nd edition (1950) *Sociologie et Anthropologie*, Presses Universitaires de France, Paris].

McArthur, M. (1977) Nutritional Research in Melanesia: A second look at the Tsembaga. In Bayliss-Smith, T. and Feachem, R. (eds) *Subsistence and Survival: rural ecology in the Pacific*, Academic Press, London: 91–128.

Mead, M. (1964) *Food Habits Research: Problems of the 1960s*, Publication 1225, National Academy of Science, National Research Council, Washington, D.C.

Mennell, S. (1985) *All manners of food: eating and taste in England and France from the Middle Ages to the present*, Blackwell, Oxford.

Museo Nacional de Antropología, España (1999) Alimentación y cultura, *Actos del Congreso Internacional 1998*, Ediciones La Val de Onsera, Huesca.

Obrist Van Eeuwijk, B. (1992) Small but strong: cultural contexts of (mal)nutrition among the Northern Kwanga (East Sepik Province, Papua New Guinea). Ethnologisches Seminar der Universität und des Museums für Völkerkunde, Basel.

Oomen, H.A.P.C. and Corden, M.W. (1970) *Metabolic Studies on New Guinean Nitrogen Metabolism in Sweet Potato Eaters*, South Pacific Commission, Technical Paper, Noumea, N° 163.

Pagézy, H. (1988) Contraintes nutritionnelles en milieu forestier équatoriel liées à la saisonnalité et la reproduction: réponses biologiques et stratégies de subsistance chez les ba-Oto et les ba-Twa du village de Nzalekenga (lac Tumba, Zaïre). *Thèse de doctorat d'Etat ès Sciences*, Université d'Aix-Marseille III.

Pelto, G., Pelto, P.J. and Messer, E. (eds) (1989) *Research Methods in Nutritional Anthropology*, The United Nations University, Tokyo.

Poulain, J.P. (2002) *Sociologies de l'Alimentation*, Presses Universitaires de France, Paris.

Rappaport, R. (1968) *Pigs for the Ancestors: ritual in the ecology of a New Guinean people,* Yale University Press, Newhaven.

Richards, A.I. (1932) *Hunger and Work in a Savage Tribe : A functional study of nutrition among the southern Bantu,* Routledge, London.

Richards, A.I. (1939) *Land, labour and diet in Northern Rhodesia: An economic study of the Bemba tribe,* Oxford University Press, London.

Richards, A.I. and Widdowson, E.M. (1936) A Dietary study in north eastern Rhodesia, *Africa,* IX(2): 166–196.

Sahlins, M.D. (1972) *Stone Age Economics,* Tavistock, London.

Simoons, J.J. (1991) *Food in China: A cultural and historical enquiry,* CRC Press, Boca Raton.

Simoons, F.J. (1994) (2nd edition, revised and enlarged) *Eat not this Flesh: food avoidance in the old world,* University of Wisconsin Press, Madison.

Steward, J.H. (1959) *Native People of South America,* MacGraw Hill, New York.

Thomas, R.B., Winterhalder, B. and McRae, S.D. (1979) An anthropological approach to human ecology and adaptive dynamics, *Yearbook of Physical Anthropology,* 22: 1–47.

Truswell, A.S. and Hansen, D.L. (1976) Medical research among the !Kung. In Lee, R.B. and de Vore, I. (eds) *Kalahari Hunter Gatherers: studies of the !Kung San and their neighbours,* Harvard University Press, Cambridge, Mass: 166–194.

Vayda, A.P. (1969) (ed.) *Environment and Cultural Behaviour,* Natural History Press, New York.

Walcher, D.N., Kretchmer, N. and Barnett, H.L. (1976) *Food, Man and Society,* Plenum Press, New York and London.

White, L.A. (1949) *The Science of Culture: A Study of Man and Civilization,* Grove Press, New York.

Wiessner, P. and Schiefenhövel, W. (eds) (1995) *Food and the Status Quest,* Berghahn Books, Oxford.

Wilson, C.S. (1979) Food Custom and Nurture: an annotated bibliography on sociocultural and biocultural aspects of nutrition, *Journal of Nutrition Education,* II(4), Supplement 1: 210–264.

Winterhalder, B. (1993) Work, resources and population in foraging societies, *Man,* 28: 321–340.

Yudkin, J. (1978) Physiological determinants of food choice. In J. Yudkin (ed.) *Diet of Man: needs and wants,* Applied Science Publishers, London: 243–260.

Yudkin, J. and McKenzie, J.C. (eds) (1964) *Changing Food Habits,* MacGibbon and Kee, London.

# 2. DEFINITIONS, CONCEPTS AND METHODS IN THE ETHNOBOTANY OF FOOD PLANTS

*Attila T. Szabó*

## Introduction

In research into the anthropology of food one should collect information from local respondents about what they eat and what are the sources for that food. This of necessity involves communication with informants about such food items. This chapter concerns the collection of data about plants used for food. In a broad sense every plant which produces substances used, raw or prepared, in human nutrition might be defined as a food plant. Indirectly, too, plants eaten by herbivores, which in turn become human food, might also be considered significant in relation to human nutrition. The basic premise for ethnobotany is that accurate communication between all concerned depends on an understanding of the nomenclature used by the local respondents, on the scientific identification of the same plants (nomenclature used by professional botanists) and on documentation for further analysis.

## Ethnobotany of Food Plants: a Neglected Field?

The primary interest in traditional human knowledge on plants is undoubtedly related to feeding and food. In spite of this, the ethnobotany of food plants is a surprisingly neglected field, as compared, for example, with the ethnobotany of plants used for medicinal purposes, or even that of the study of plant names. One of the reasons for this perhaps is that knowledge about food plants gradually became a part, but only a part, of many different scientific fields, such as agrobotany (e.g. Simmonds 1976, Hanelt *et al.* 2001), gastronomy, pharmacobotany, etc. Food plant ethnobotany is also integrated into the social sciences (Wiessner and Schiefenhövel 1995), and into the food sciences (e.g. Owen 1990, Bérard *et al.* 1993). Furthermore it is a favourite subject for popular sciences (Vickery 1997). Too many cooks spoiled the broth. Perhaps only a new, multidisciplinary approach will bring the strands together again.

## Aims and Definitions

### Aims

The main aim of this chapter is to present some basic definitions, concepts and methods of food *ethnobotany*, which may influence data collection and analysis. Some problems related to scientific and folk nomenclature and classifications are discussed and examples which underline the importance of infraspecific variability in food plants are given. As well, some guidelines regarding the herbarium documentation needed for laboratory work are outlined.

### The Evolution of Definitions

Ethnobotany includes a wide range of possible approaches and consequently has many possible definitions. According to the original North American approach (Harshberger 1896, Davis 1995), ethnobotany is the study of plant use and of 'botanical' knowledge accumulated in *primitive, indigenous* and *aboriginal* societies, as opposed to 'economic botany', which is about plant use and related knowledge in advanced agro-industrial societies (Schultes and Reis 1995, Turner 1995). The basic problem with this definition resides in the meaning of the words *primitive, indigenous* and *aboriginal*, used instead of a word suggesting traditional folk use. Even though the ethnobotany of traditional societies with less advanced technology remains an important part of this field of study (Anderson 1993, Prance 1995, Prance *et al.* 1995), food plant use in 'modern' societies also has important traditional, ethnobotanical components almost everywhere in the world. In Europe, including central Europe which is now interrelating increasingly with the European Union, there are large indigenous populations which retain a good traditional knowledge about food plants.

European ethnobotany has a long history rooted deeply in different national or ethnic traditions, but also in mediaeval and renaissance European herbalism (Arber 1938). This herbalism produced the first independent printed books with ethnobotanical and ethnomycological data, including information on food plants and *fungi* (Clusius and Beythe 1583, Clusius 1603 cf. Szabó 1978, Szabó *et al.* 1992). Renaissance herbalism, which is derived mostly from Greek, Roman, Judaeo-Christian (biblical) and local folk traditions, flourished during the sixteenth century and may be regarded as a transition between traditional and scientific botany. In herbalism, oral ethnobotanical knowledge was slowly merged into organised science. Herbalists gradually recognised the value of natural biological categories (genera and species in a pre-Linnaean sense) creating the basis for scientific nomenclature. They also preserved in their writings ethnobotanical categories (folk names and knowledge) in European science for centuries. Ethnobotany is still essential for understanding the origin and evolution of plant names in different languages.

The ethnobotany of the enigmatic Lapp people, encountered by Carl von Linné (also known as Linnaeus) during a journey in Lappland in 1732, was one of the starting points for the 'Linnaean Revolution' (Linné 1753). Linné was the first to separate ethnobotany completely from scientific botany and his sexual system and binominal nomenclature of species dominated the scientific view until the new evolutionary species paradigm, propounded by Charles Darwin in 1859 and 1868, gained acceptance. In the middle of the twentieth century another shift of paradigm followed the discovery of the chemical structure of DNA as a primary source of biological information. Another shift is in progress now with the advent of genomics. The first full plant genome sequence (the *Arabidopsis* genome) was published on 14th December, 2000 in *Nature*, London (n.c.). New molecular studies of the nature of taxonomic categories contribute indirectly to a better understanding of some ethnobotanical categories such as local and/or regional traditional cultivars (land races).

The Linnaean and even the Darwinian periods were notable in plant sciences for their general rejection of oral ethnobotanical knowledge. Beginning with the middle of the twentieth century, however, ethnobotany has become increasingly respected as a science which supports sustainability, organic farming, etc. It is regarded as an interdisciplinary field focused on the study of orally transmitted botanical knowledge from different ethnic and/or cultural communities (Szabó and Péntek 1976, Schultes and Reis 1995, Vickery 1997, etc.). The collection of plant material, suited for resource conservation and reproduction (genetic resources) and for traditional knowledge connected mainly with food, is also included in this approach (e.g. Vavilov 1992[1932], Balick and Cox 1996, Hammer 1998, I. Szabó *et al.* 2000, Hanelt *et al.* 2001).

Global changes (and indirectly the *Man and Biosphere* programme followed by the biodiversity conservation projects launched in Rio de Janeiro, 1960–1992, 1992–2002 n.c.) and the recognition of genetic diversity as a base of infraspecific variability gradually led to a reconsideration of ethnobotany (e.g. Hladik *et al.* 1990). In the process, ethnobotany came to be reconsidered and accepted as the study of general relationships between plants and people, and of the interactions between local people and the natural environment in any cultural community. In this approach ethnobotany is a part of ethnoecological (Péntek and Szabó 1985, Martin 1995) or ethnobiodiversity studies (Szabó *et al.* 1992, Szabó and Pentek 1996, Szabó 1999, 2002). This new tendency is connected with new phenomena in the history of science: environmentalism, sustainability, biodiversity protection, globalisation, and the growing gap between the scientific (organised, computerised, molecular, etc.) knowledge and the traditional, orally transmitted knowledge of plants.

## Scientific and Folk Taxonomy and Food Ethnobotany

One basic problem in the ethnobotany of food plants resides in the difference between scientific and folk taxonomy. Both are linked by the human urge to group, name and understand the diversity of nature and the diversity of organisms observed in the environment: a 'taxonomic' urge. Both scientific and folk taxonomies are based on a selected set of similarities and differences, but scientific classifications are supported by formal analysis rather better than oral classifications are. *Ethnotaxonomy* is pragmatic (e.g.'edible' *versus* 'inedible'), but also generally irrational in that it has no logical cause-and-effect explications. The need to understand the origin of variability in plants (including food plants) is limited to scientific taxonomy and evolutionary botany.

*Scientific Taxonomy* provides a continuously evolving logical system for the classification of different organisms, based on rules of nomenclature and systematics. Scientific nomenclature is focused on rules of naming. Systematics deal with the practice of grouping the units behind the names. Names are essential for exploration of the environment. We are generally unable to memorise and handle large sets of numbers, but we handle large sets of names more easily.

A living unit of nature, once named scientifically, is called a *taxon*. In botanical science a *taxon* is based on the concept of typification (i.e. every higher taxonomical category is based on well-defined lower ranked types). Plant *taxa* are thus organised in a hierarchical system. In contrast, a folk taxonomy is utilitarian: it is based on practical considerations, it is not hierarchical, has no typification, but has its own reason based often on scientifically ungrounded beliefs.

The basic unit in scientific taxonomy is the *species*. The species concept is deeply rooted in European science today. It was defined formally first by Linné (Linné 1753), based on morphological similarity, reproductive isolation and a concept of separate divine creation. This concept of species has been succeeded over the last 250 years by a series of 'new' concepts of evolutionary species, making the category highly controversial. More than twenty different, mostly mutually exclusive, definitions of species are now considered in the literature on the topic (Hey 2001). The picture is further complicated by even more controversial infraspecific categories, as shown by the vegetable and fruit examples given below [*Brassica* (cabbage), *Phaseolus* (bean), *Beta* (beetroot) and *Prunus* (plum)].

The practice of botanical taxonomy (nomenclature and systematics) is a carefully regulated process. The scientific, botanical nomenclature has, in theory, universal acceptance. The ethnobotanical (vernacular) nomenclature, i.e. the folk nomenclature in the broadest sense, is the traditional way of naming different plant groups. It is not regulated by written rules and has a restricted local or regional acceptance. The system of official plant names in any national language (folk nomenclature in a restricted sense) represents a transition between the two, because now the folk nomenclature *sensu stricto* is more or less standardised in many languages and is often correlated with the scientific nomenclature.

*Synonymy* (different names for the same unit) and *homonymy* (the same name for different units) are frequent in both scientific and folk taxonomy, even in the same language. Global language diversity makes folk taxonomy not only a really exciting topic, but also essential for research into the anthropology of food.

The stability of both scientific and folk taxonomies is relative. Scientific taxonomy is relatively stable across space (e.g. across languages and cultures), while some folk names have remained the same or very similar for centuries, but each only in its own local, regional, and social context. That is to say, folk names tend to be restricted in space but quite stable over time. In contrast, the corresponding scientific names may have changed frequently for scientific (evolutionary) or even non-scientific reasons (e.g. vanity). For example the scientific nomenclature for wheat grasses (included in *Triticum, Agropyron, Elymus, Leymus, Elytrigia* and many other genera) has been constantly changing at genus and species levels over the last couple of centuries, while the folk nomenclature remained quite constant (at least in some languages). The situation is similar for many other *taxa*.

A striking example of conceptual differences between folk and scientific taxonomy can be found in the genus *Brassica* (cabbage family). The domestication of the wild cabbage (*Brassica oleracea*) caused a spectacular evolution in forms, functions and use of different plant parts. This is also reflected in the vernacular names of different *taxa*, which sound quite unrelated. Only the scientific names express the underlying evolutionary relationship between them all (Table 2.1).

***Table 2.1*** Conceptual differences between scientific and folk taxonomies: the *Brassica* case

| Scientific category (*taxon*) | Vernacular names | Scientific synonymy |
|---|---|---|
| *Brassica olearcea* var. *acephala* | kale, collards, *borecole | |
| – – var. *alboglabra* | chinese kale | *B. alboglabra* |
| – – var. *borytis* | **broccoli, cauliflower | |
| – – var. *capitata* | cabbage, savoy cabbage | |
| – – var. *chinensis* | pak-choi | *B. chinensis* |
| – – var. *costata* | tronchuda (-kale, -cabagge) | *B. o.* var. *tronchuda* |
| – – var. *gemmifera* | Brussels-sprouts | |
| – – var. *gongylodes* | Kohlrabi | *B. caulorapa* |
| – – var. *italica* | Sprouting (asparagus) **broccoli | |
| – – var. *pekinensis* | chinese cabbage, celery cabbage | *B. pekinensis* |

*: similar vernacular names (possibility of confusion)
**: homonyms (danger of confusion)

In the case of *Phaseolus* (beans), the infraspecific taxonomy based on characteristics caused by 'marker' genes acting on seed form, size, colour and seed coat pattern is widely used for differentiating between varieties according their nutritive, gastronomic and culinary values. The same is true for the fruit characteristics in the *Prunus* species (plums, cherries, apricots, almonds, etc.) or the root characteristics as is the case for *Beta* species (beetroots) (Péntek and Szabó 1985).

So, it is important to emphasise again and again that the categories used in folk taxonomy differ from those used in scientific taxonomy. For this reason there is no perfect correlation between the two. It is wise to keep this in mind during fieldwork, and even more importantly during the analysis of the results. There is no 'genus-level' and 'species-level' ranking in ethnotaxonomy.


## How to Collect Information

*Collection.* Basic methods in the field of food ethnobotany are the same as those used in general qualitative and quantitative ethnobotanical studies. The main goal here is to focus interest on food plants. So, women directly involved in work with food for the family will be preferred as informants. However, complementary information is also needed from men, children and the elderly (see also Hubert, this volume). Notes on age, ethnicity, religion, origin (place of birth), place of childhood, age at marriage, kinship, family size, family structure, number of generations in the household, occupation, social status, literacy, education, language abilities and migration records should ideally also be recorded for every informant/respondent, if research time allows.

If informants are chosen randomly, the result will be more representative of the general situation, but this is not always practicable. If the most informative members of the population are selected as respondents, the data collected will be more comprehensive, but possibly less characteristic of the general situation. It should be remembered that both the verbal and the non-verbal behaviour of the researcher may influence the results. Language skills (talking the language of the informant), mutual respect, confidentiality (keeping secrets) and many other personal skills are important for successful fieldwork. If time is not a primary limiting factor, *participant observation* (PO) in the field, in the market, in the kitchen, at the dining table etc. and a carefully maintained ethnobotanical field diary are important for the collection of information. PO is the most useful method for discovering details and understanding causal relations.

*Open-ended conversations* (OEC), e.g. joint walks in crop fields, home gardens, but also more generally in forests and meadows, etc., also tend to reveal interesting knowledge with many unexpected details. However, totally unstructured OECs also bear a high risk of omission of important facts. Many omissions can be avoided using *semi-structured interviews* (SSI), following a list of questions and using a set of well-selected pictures of food plants prepared beforehand. Using SSIs all questions considered important are covered. Moreover, they are asked in a logical order and recorded systematically in the case of every respondent. This method has great advantages during the analysis and synthesis of the results. SSIs do not exclude, of course, free flowing conversations on related or unrelated topics as one goes along.

If time is strictly limited and the aim is a systematic survey of every important question in different social, ethnic, rural, religious or age communities, a *fully structured interview* system may be followed, although this has the risk of formality, which may be less attractive or even disturbing and exhausting for the informant.

Differences in gender, age, religion, clothing, cultural backgrounds, empathy, etc. between respondents and the interviewers may affect the collection of good data. For example, a properly dressed woman scientist belonging to the same cultural community will perhaps work more effectively with local women informants. The results will of course also depend upon many other interpersonal skills. Furthermore, the results will be different working in private (i.e. one interviewer with one respondent) from working in groups. In the latter case, a further diversity of situations may occur when working with homogenous or with heterogenous groups of respondents, and whether these are faced by a single researcher or by a group of interviewers. Our practice (Szabó and Péntek 1976, Péntek and Szabó 1985) is for a team of two, a botanist-geneticist and a linguist-ethnographer to work together. This has proved to be very effective.

*Interviews* may be limited to a single occasion, or repeated several times at different intervals with different groups. In the case of PO the event may be continuous for a period, but for other studies the information sought may cover several different periods; for example when a group of local school children is asked about their daily food intake during different seasons of the year. Furthermore, research should not focus only on plant *taxa* and recipes, which simply results in qualitative lists, but should also go into their relative abundance and into the preferences of the respondents. This provides the opportunity for a more effective analysis.

*Quantitative ethnobotanical analysis*: Traditional ethnobotany was, and still is, largely descriptive, that is *qualitative*. It rarely adventures into the field of numerical analysis and hypothesis testing. Apart from historical reasons, this is partly explained by the difficulties in collecting and evaluating numerical data gathered during complex and often incoherent ethnobotanical fieldwork. Participant observation and open-ended discussions are not suited for the collection of numerical data. It was not until the second half of the twentieth century that laboratory and field methods were developed in order to collect numerical data which allow a quantitative (numerical) analysis of the qualitative aspects of ethnobotanical data, using, for example, preference ranking, direct matrix ranking, paired comparisons, triadic comparisons, pile sorting, etc.

## Documenting Information

## Botanical Documentation: an Ethnobotanical Herbarium on Food Plant Diversity

The differences between scientific, vernacular and folk taxonomy, and the familial, local, regional, cultural and ethnic/linguistic peculiarities in naming plant varieties, belonging to the same species, are good reasons why collection of a herbarium is strongly recommended during research. Food plant ethnobotany is often concerned with infraspecific taxonomy. Exact identification of such small intraspecific differences is rarely possible in the field. So, specimens need to be taken to a laboratory. For laboratory and/or experimental studies good herbarium samples, clear photographs or even living collections are needed for identification, evaluation and/or *ex situ* cultivation or conservation. Good herbarium specimens, prepared even by the simplest means (e.g. pressed and dried between newspaper pages), numbered and labelled with year/ month/day/hour/minute on every label (as well as any labelling for customs requirements) should be noted exactly in the field notebook. This later allows a more sure and detailed taxonomical identification. The scientific value of the fieldwork, and of the time and money spent on it, is greatly increased by these simple means. Without correct identification the collected data can be misleading and would have no or limited value.

## Audio-visual and Written Documentation: Pictures, Audio and Video Tapes, Field Notes

Digital photographs, labelled and numbered automatically with year/month/ day/hour/minute inscriptions, allow a good correlation with well labelled herbarium and/or living plant or seed collections, as well as with the field notes, audio and video tapes. In the first phase, during the fieldwork, using all these modern techniques may be disturbing both for interviewers and respondents. Whatever else is used or not, the field notes provide the basic documentation which is essential. In the second phase, in the laboratory, the time available is the limiting factor, as identification, rewriting, control and database building is a time consuming process. Even so, material gathered by modern techniques, where possible, is of great assistance in the second, laboratory phase.

## Analysis and Dissemination of the Data

## Analysis

Qualitative data presented in the form of lists are analysed in a traditional way. Quantitative data collected from structured interviews can be analysed numerically after arrangement in a matrix. Numerical results can be tested for significance, according to the objectives and needs of the study in progress. If different collections follow the same protocol, the results will allow better comparisons, hypothesis-testing and the formulation of firmer conclusions.

A simple *preference ranking*, for example, allows one to compare a fixed number of items arranged by every respondent in her/his order of preference (with highest values given to the most preferred items). Such a matrix will have the general form shown in Table 2.2. Starting from this very simple example, different matrix tables can be constructed with preferred *taxa*, preferred characteristics, preferences in paired and triadic comparisons or with in-pile sorting (the division of objects into groups according to the similarity of certain features). Working with a sufficient number of respondents this should allow the production of comparable, significant results. This is the way that qualitative, descriptive food ethnobotany can be transformed into quantitative, causal food ethnobotany, as will be required for ethnobiodiversity studies in the third Millennium.

From a well balanced and sufficiently large sample one may calculate the preference ranking of different criteria (e.g. *taxon* or characteristics) at individual respondent, group and/or community levels.

***Table 2.2*** Preference ranking: example of an ethnobotanical matrix comparing preferences based on a number of criteria (*taxon*, characteristics, etc.) arranged by every respondent according to his or her order of preference

| Respondent | Preference value (best is the highest) | | | | | |
|---|---|---|---|---|---|---|
| | 1st Criterion | 2nd Criterion | 3rd Criterion | 4th Criterion | N Criterion | Mean/ respondent |
| 1st | 2 | 4 | 1 | 3 | | |
| 2nd | 3 | 4 | 1 | 2 | | |
| 3rd | 4 | 3 | 2 | 1 | | |
| 4th | 4 | 3 | 1 | 2 | | |
| N Respondent Mean | 3.25 | 3.50 | 1.25 | 2.25 | | |

## Synthesis

Analysis does not end with the production of the figures, calculations, tables, etc. The results must be described and reviewed, and conclusions drawn in the full text of the written papers.

## Dissemination

There are now two basic possibilities for dissemination of the results:

1. to publish a traditionally organised, ethnobotanical paper or mono-
   graph, or
2. to publish on a simple or 'interactive' site on the Internet.

The traditional, conservative solution of publication in academic, peer-
reviewed literature seems the best way to conserve the results, and allows a
sound citation basis for the author. But it is often expensive, time consuming
and does not, in fact, allow free and worldwide availability of all data. The
modern electronic way of publishing is supported now by a number of different, sophisticated computer systems and programs. Results can be published
with or without peer review on the Internet or on a CD-ROM with all the
advantages and disadvantages of this kind of publication. The peer-reviewed
possibility of e-publication emerged between 1990 and 2000, but this author's
own experience of electronic publication in 1990, 1996, 2000 and 2001 (refer-
ences not cited here), both in Internet and in CD-ROM format, revealed high
risks in this method of dissemination.

A well designed, functional, Internet-based *Comparative International Electronic Ethnobotanical Database* is still a dream.

## Concluding Remarks

Food plants were and are of primordial importance, but the ethnobotany of
food is still a methodologically weak and relatively neglected research field.
The subject of food ethnobotany depends largely on definitions adopted for
ethnobotany as a science. Defined in a narrow sense, food plant ethnobotany
is limited to 'traditional' societies. Defined in a broad sense, the ethnobotany
of food is relevant for any cultural community, as a cross-disciplinary field of
study between the arts (culinary art) and the biological and the social sciences,
involving different (sub)fields of botany, anthropology/ethnography, nutritional sciences, etc. While most of the work to date has been qualitative in style,
the quantitative ethnobotany of food plants is a promising field for the future.

However, it is clear that researchers into the anthropology of food, especially in cultures different from their own, must have at least the limited introduction to ethnobotany provided in this chapter, because correlating the folk
taxonomy to the scientific taxonomy is a basic requirement for identification
of plants used in foods. Without proper identification many of the subsequent
uses of the descriptive material, such as for the estimation of nutrients or for
comparison with other populations, will be lost.

The cross-disciplinary cooperation of different specialists is again strongly
recommended in this endeavour.

## Acknowledgements

The author acknowledges the generous help of Helen Macbeth, co-editor of this volume, for her very useful suggestions and corrections.

## References

Anderson, E. (1993) *Plants and People of the Golden Triangle*, Discorides Press, Portland.

Arber, A. (1938) *Herbals, their Origin and Evolution*, Cambridge University Press, Cambridge.

Balick, M.J. and Cox, P.A. (1996) *Plants, People, and Culture: The Science of Ethnobotany*, Scientific American Library, New York.

Berard, L., Froc, J., Hyman, M., Hyman, P. and Marchenay, P. (1993) *Ile-de-France: Produits du terroir*, Conseil National des Arts Culinaires, Paris.

Clusius, C. (1583, 1584): *Stirpium per Pannoniam, Austriam* etc., Plantin, Antverpen.

Clusius, C. and St. B(eythe) (1583, 1584): *Stirpium Nomenclator Pannonicus*, Manlius, Németújvár, (1583), Plantin, Antverpen.

Davis, E.A. (1995) Ethnobotany: an old practice, a new discipline. In Schultes, R.E. and Reis, S.von (eds) *Ethnobotany: Evolution of a discipline*, Dioscorides Press, Portland, Oregon: 40–51.

Hammer, K. (1998) *Agrobiodiversität und pflanzengenetischen Ressourcen – Herausförderung und Lösungsatz*. Schriften zu Genetischen Resourcen, Bd. 10, Informationszentrum für Genetische Ressourcen, Zentralstelle für Agrardokumentation und -information, Bonn.

Hanelt, P. and Institute of Plant Genetics and Crop Plant Research (eds) (2001) *Mansfeld's Encyclopedia of Agricultural and Horticultural Crops*. Springer, Berlin vols. 1–6.

Harshberger, J.W. (1896) Purposes of ethnobotany, *Botanical Gazette* 21(3): 146–154.

Hey, J. (2001) The mind of the species problem, *Trends in Ecology and Evolution*, 16(7): 327.

Hladik, C.M., Bahuchet S. and Garine I.de, (eds)(1990) *Food and Nutrition in the African Rain Forest*, UNESCO/Man and Biosphere, Paris.

Linné, C. von (1753) *Species plantarum*. Stockholm.

Martin, G.J. (1995) *Ethnobotany: A methods manual*, Chapman and Hall, London.

Owen, F.D. (1990) *The Plants We Eat*. In Chapman, M. and Macbeth, H. (eds) *Food for Humanity: cross-disciplinary readings*, Centre for the Sciences of Food and Nutrition, Oxford: 63–71.

Péntek, J. and Szabó, T.A. (1985) *Ember és növényvilág. Kalotaszeg növényzete és népi növényismerete. (Man and the Plant World. Plant Kingdom and Traditional Human Life)*. Kriterion, Bucharest.

Prance, G.T. (1995) Ethnobotany Today and in the Future. In Schultes, R.E. and Reis, S.von (eds) *Ethnobotany: evolution of a discipline*, Dioscorides Press, Portland, Oregon: 60–68.

Prance, G.T., Balée, W., Boom, B.M. and Carneiro, L.R. (1995) Quantitative Ethnobotany and the Case for Conservation in Amazonia. In Schultes, R.E. and Reis, S.von (eds) *Ethnobotany: evolution of a discipline*, Dioscorides Press, Portland, Oregon: 157–174.

Schultes, R.E. and Reis, S.von, (eds)(1995) *Ethnobotany: evolution of a discipline,* Dioscorides Press, Portland, Oregon.

Simmonds, N.W. (ed.)(1976) *Evolution of Crop Plants,* Longman, London.

Szabó, I., Grynaeus T. and. Szabó L.Gy., (2000) *The role of ethnobotany in the evaluation of agrobiodiversity* (in Hungarian). In Gyulai, F. (ed.) *Preservation and Use of Agrobiodiversity: Proceedings dedicated to A. Jánossy (1908–1975), the founder of the Hungarian Agrobotanical Institute and Genebank,* Agricultural Museum (Budapest) and the Institute of Agrobotany (Tápiószele): 249–255.

Szabó, T.A. (ed.)(1978) *Melius Péter: Herbarium (1578),* Kriterion, Bucharest.

Szabó, T.A. (1999) Genetic Erosion, Human Environment and Ethnobiodiversity Studies. In Serwinski, J. and Faberová, I. (eds) *Proceedings of the Technical Meeting on the Methodology of the FAO World Information and Early Warning System on Plant Genetic Resources,* FAO Research Institute for Crop Production, Prague: 76–83.

Szabó, T.A. (in press), *Ethnobotanical studies on cultivated plants. A theoretical approach. Studies on Ethnobiodiversity (6). Proceedings of the Symposium "Rudolf Mansfeld and Plant Genetic Resources",* Institute für Kulturpflanzenforschung Gatersleben.

Szabó, T.A. and Péntek J. (1976) *Centaurium: Ethnobotanical Guide Book* (in Hungarian), first edition, Kriterion, Bucharest; [second edition, Tankönyv-kiadó, Budapest (1996)].

Szabó, T.A., Szabó, I. and Wolkinger, F. (eds)(1992) *The Beginnings of Pannonian Ethnobotany: Stirpium Nomenclator Pannonicus edited by S(tephanus) B(eythe) (1583), Carolus Clusius (1583/84), David Czvittinger (1711).* Steinamanger – Graz – Güssing. Collecta Clusiana, 2: 1–142.

Turner, N.J. (1995) Ethnobotany Today in Northwestern North America. In Schultes, R.E. and Reis S.von, (eds) *Ethnobotany: evolution of a discipline,* Dioscorides Press, Portland, Oregon: 264–283.

Vavilov, N.I. (1992[1932]) *Origin and Geography of Cultivated Plants.* (D. Löve, translation.), Cambridge University Press, Cambridge.

Vickery, R. (1997) *A Dictionary of Plant-Lore.* Oxford University Press, Oxford.

Wiessner, P. and Schiefenhövel, W. (1995) *Food and the Status Quest: an interdisciplinary perspective,* Berghahn, Oxford.

Also, the following websites may be useful:

* *http://binet-biotar.vein.hu* (BioTár Electronic: Amplicon, Collecta Clusiana).
* *http://mansfeld.ipk-gatersleben.de* (Mansfeld Database of Cultivated Plants).

# 3. QUALITATIVE RESEARCH IN THE ANTHROPOLOGY OF FOOD
## A COMPREHENSIVE QUALITATIVE/QUANTITATIVE APPROACH

*Annie Hubert*

## Introduction

The quarrel about choosing between quantitative and qualitative research should be obsolete. A comprehensive method should combine both, especially in the field of anthropology of food where both approaches exist, have often been divergent, but ideally should be combined.

One of the first anthropologists to have thought seriously about methods in collecting food-related data was Margaret Mead, acting for the Department of State of the United States of America, during the Second World War. On rereading her manual, it is surprising to see that it has not aged at all, and that the methods she suggests are still those we would use today (Mead 1945). She already recommended that quantitative nutritional research should be combined with qualitative social science and psychological data on food habits.

All food-related research, from the most basic nutritional data to food symbolism, behaviour and beliefs, needs to be placed in its proper background or context in order to be coherent. Indeed, this is what Mead insisted upon. Food being a central activity of all living beings, and a particularly complex activity among humans, requires an approach which will do justice to all the intertwined themes and structures which construct human social and biological behaviour related to food. Methods should be combined for a completely holistic approach.

## Defining the Aims of a Study

The first and most important methodological step is to be quite clear about the proposed aims of a study.

## 1. What Group of People are you Going to be Working on?

The anthropological problem of defining a 'population' arises here. The possibilities are numerous: a small community of people living in a same area, a particular socio-economic or professional group, a particular age group, only women, or only men, a large population in a culturally defined area, or indeed a whole nation.

## 2. What Particular Aspect of Food and Food Ways Should be Studied?

This could be the assessment of nutritional status, or the description of the diet of a population and the various strategies used to have access to food. It could also be concerned with all the technical processes of storing and transforming food, or with cuisine as a means of expression, or it could focus more specifically on food-related behaviour, on food beliefs and symbols, on consumer attitudes, preferences, on food as an economic issue, on diet-related diseases, on issues of public health and food hygiene, and so on. There is a great diversity of possible aspects to study, but in all cases the focus chosen will condition the first step in gathering available data.

## 3. What is the Framework?

Once the aims have been defined, the material gathered has still to be set within an appropriate framework. It makes no sense to study nutrition in minute detail if one does not know where the food comes from, what the individuals do with it, how they eat it and when. Researchers need to know, not only what people eat, but how and why they eat that way as well. The very nature of food studies means that each investigator will broach a network of related themes even if the primary focus of the study seems at first quite narrow.

## Preliminary Basic Information

As in any other academic venture, a survey of existing literature on the chosen area is necessary. Nutritionists, sociologists, anthropologists and psychologists have all written on the theme of food in many areas, in both industrialised and developing countries. Also, there may well be studies of women's and food magazines, local cookbooks, food advertisements, etc. Quantitative nutritional surveys, if they exist for the defined population, should be consulted, as should all epidemiological studies relating to food intake. Local or national statistics on food consumption and food production are also very helpful. All these readings help in the design of the study and in the formulation of research hypotheses. This first bibliographical step is essential and it is worthwhile spending considerable time on it.

## Which Approach for Which Study?

In this chapter the advice is that a qualitative approach is beneficial as a preliminary part of the research, even when the ultimate aim is to conduct a quantitative study. It saves both money and time. Whatever the study, a *three-step strategy* combining both qualitative and quantitative methods should produce adequate and reliable data. Since this chapter is mainly concerned with qualitative methods for food-related research, the necessary steps required for quantitative data will be given less attention.

## Step I – Surveying Existing Data

Whenever possible, even with qualitative research methods, one should begin by studying existing descriptive and quantitative data on food consumption. These can be found through national statistics, consumer surveys, certain nutritional surveys, as well as in the literature mentioned above, and they may help, among other things, to define specific groupings of people within the study population.

Quantitative epidemiological data can also be very useful for defining geographical areas, marked differences in food-related pathologies and general nutritional status. Economic data can give further general information on food consumption, food production and distribution. This kind of background information is essential for the study.

## Step II – Anthropological Qualitative Study

Although it is only an introductory 'step', its description is the main topic of this chapter. For it is qualitative data which provide the background and the context of any food-related study. It is well worthwhile spending a good deal of time on it, since in the end it will provide a better focus for the collection of quantitative information and so reduce the time and the expenses of this.

When the aims of a study have been well defined, the type of population chosen, and general data on the topic collected and reviewed, the serious business of collecting qualitative data can start.

## A Small Representative Group

What is needed is a group of people with whom one can carry out detailed fieldwork. Unlike most nutritional studies, anthropological ones deal with households or family groups. An individual is part of a social group composed of various different units and his or her behaviour is conditioned by this social and cultural environment. An investigator can only obtain any reasonable understanding of this environment, and thus of local behaviours and beliefs, by including whole household units within the data collection. This holds true even for studies particularly concerned with individual behaviour and health status.

One has to start with a specific definition of the local 'family unit' or household. In North European countries it can be the nuclear family and its related groups including single parent households. In other areas it can be the extended families of whatever type. A good definition and description are needed.

In field research on food in Europe or elsewhere, we need to know how different generations communicate and live: together, separately, with or without contact. Food-related behaviour and beliefs are never static. Food systems are dynamic. To describe and understand the context, we need to observe two or three generations, in order to bring to light various transmission processes on food and food ways. This family 'background' is just as important if the group for study is defined by a specific description of person, e.g. obese, with nutritional disorders, diabetics, etc. In all cases, the relationship within the family group will influence behaviour, choices and preferences.

For the statistical purposes of further quantitative studies, the minimum number required is thirty and this thirty or more has to be representative of the chosen population. This is where socio-economic and epidemiological data come in. The sample can be chosen using a 'network' system: once the socio-economic and age profiles of the general population are known, you start by picking one household unit belonging to a specific category, and by asking its members if they know of another household belonging to another particular profile; you meet another, ask again, and so on. You continue like this until you have completed the sample of thirty households, including, where possible, two-adult-generation households, covering all the predefined, socio-economic, professional or other required types. In other words, according to local circumstances, the survey can be made up of fifteen families, if each comprises two nuclear groups of different generations. Then, representativeness is ensured.

# Fieldwork

What follows is social anthropological style of fieldwork, and it requires three basic techniques:

## 1. Participant Observation

The researcher establishes relations with the families, and chooses either to spend some weeks or months in their vicinity, allowing for daily or nearly daily visits, or lives within one of these households, or manages to travel every day to his or her 'field'. This will enable the fieldworker to observe and describe the habitat, in our case mainly the kitchen, cooking facilities and instruments of the families, to observe the storage conditions and purchase of goods, to accompany members of the household to shops and/or gardens, to observe in situ the cooking activities and ideally to share the meals as well. All this is noted in a notebook coded for the family unit. It is recommended that notes are written up as soon as possible and certainly within twenty-four hours. This visual observation is a necessary addition to the data obtained through questions and conversations.

If time is an issue, not all thirty households need to be approached in this way, but at least six should be surveyed in this manner.

## 2. Non-directed or Semi-directed Interviews

Informal exchange and conversations are the basis of good qualitative data recording. The fieldworker should note in their notebook all relevant information which might have come up in general conversations. Conversations should be held with the person in charge of cooking and/or shopping. They should be informal, and recorded. The person or persons recorded should be allowed free conversation on food. The notebook should be labelled with the appropriate identification code.

In addition, semi-directed interviews covering predetermined topics should be carried out with key members of the household, i.e. those who cook and the elderly for past memories. The easiest technique is to establish an interview guide, such as the one presented as an appendix to this chapter. Interviews should be recorded. Be sure that the audio tape is labelled with name, number and date, and this information written in a 'field journal' where daily field events are noted. The guide is there mainly as a reminder of all the aspects to be covered. It helps later analysis if each time one more or less follows the same structure as in that guide. The recordings then are completely transcribed, and kept in separate files for each family group, coded and labelled in the same way as the notebooks. It helps to transcribe the audio tapes as one goes along, rather than wait until all fieldwork has been completed. It is less tedious and also allows one to develop new queries as the fieldwork develops.

### 3. Life Histories

It does seem peculiar to insist on collecting life histories for food-related research. However, we find it very revealing of beliefs, transformations, transmissions, etc.; it gives an even more solid context and background to contemporary studies. The older people are recorded, telling the 'food story' of their lives, including the transformations in the way of acquiring and transforming foods.

## Analysis

Qualitative analysis tends to frighten those used to the mathematical formulas of quantitative studies. Content analysis does not need to be over complicated. It all depends on the number of 'files' to analyse. In this case, thirty files, one per family group, is not an impossible task and does not require heavy and difficult computer programs. A manual system can be handy: chop up the recorded conversations into packages of themes and give them a number and sub- number by family. Thus you might have 'Interview family 1, A (older generation) and B (younger)', in which each theme would be separated. Put together all separate themes with their identification codes, and you have your analysis nearly done. All you have to do is read, count and think. You will come up with things like 'more than half the family groups have dinner together in the evening', or 'three out of thirty groups never go to the market'. You can develop observations such as 'the younger generations eat less animal fat than the older', and so on. In this way you will have accumulated detailed data on foods obtained, how they are obtained, how they are cooked and when they are eaten. You will also know what people think about health and diet, how and why they purchase food stuffs, and how they deal with children and food: in other words, all the immaterial aspects of social life surrounding food and food behaviour.

Chopping up the texts, grouping them, analysing the contents is lengthy but worthwhile. The understanding that one gains at the end is a seemingly comprehensive context, a solid background, on to which later quantitative data can be applied for various types of study. This 'Step II' allows space for informed thought before setting up a well-constructed study using a questionnaire. In many research areas, such as for themes covering nutritional epidemiology, hypotheses formulated for quantitative testing are greatly improved when based on detailed, qualitative data, as described above.

## Step III – Quantifying to Test the Qualitative Results

As already pointed out, the qualitative data provides information necessary for formulating a very complete and easily coded questionnaire on food habits, designed for a specific group in a specific area and covering all the detailed information on foods, recipes, types of dishes, frequencies as well as beliefs and types of behaviour. It is important to stress that the design of the questionnaire should be done with the collaboration of statisticians so as to obtain the easiest design for later quantitative analysis. Statisticians have methods for quantitative analysis which will not be discussed in this chapter

## Quantifying to Test Specific Hypotheses

The specific hypotheses may be related to social conditions, nutritional status, epidemiology, public health or market research, or they may confirm the earlier qualitative research with a larger data set. Collaboration with the relevant specialists is likely already to exist and is, of course, necessary. The earlier qualitative data is analysed to identify specific types of behaviour leading to the establishment of hypotheses. For example, if one is working on a population of diabetics, the qualitative data might have identified a specific popular belief about the effect of sugar in the diet. This could lead to a well formulated question in the questionnaire to see if the belief did actually affect the health status of the whole population. Questionnaires, therefore, must be individually designed for the hypothesis under consideration.

## Comparative Studies

Comparing data on two, or more, generations in each household will assist the understanding of the dynamics of change in food and diet, since one should always bear in mind that the relationship between humans and their food is part of a system of perpetual transformation.

Comparative studies are particularly interesting when they combine nutritional epidemiology and anthropology. When researching, for example, dietary factors associated with certain types of disease, an anthropological qualitative study, such as described above, carried out within two distinct populations, could lead to useful comparative analysis. The differences in diet would then show up; these would enable the formulation of food factor hypotheses, which could then be tested quantitatively by case control studies using a simple questionnaire.

Conversely, two distinct populations showing the same epidemiological risk for a certain disease could be compared through an anthropological qualitative study for similarities in diet. This could then lead to well formulated hypotheses about food-related risk factors. An example of this method is a study on nasopharyngeal cancer and dietary factors (Hubert 1990, Hubert *et al.* 1992).

## Applying the Questionnaire

The ideal situation is for the questionnaires, whether individual or for a household, to be filled in by an investigator in the home and, if possible, in the presence of the individual respondent or the whole household group. This sort of information tends to be more precise, but it takes a long time.

Questionnaires may be sent by post to individuals to fill in. This method is often used by sociologists and others, as a very large number of participants can be reached. However, there is no way to judge the accuracy of the information given and bias can exist in those who respond (Macbeth *et al.* 2002).

## Conclusion

In this chapter, a three-step approach to research into food-related behaviour has been recommended:

1. A general gathering of information on a chosen population before undertaking fieldwork;
2. A qualitative anthropological field study on a small sample of that population, preferably including two generations of adults;
3. The qualitative data is then used to set up a questionnaire to produce quantitative data on a larger population sample. Analysis of the quantitative data may be used simply to confirm the qualitative study using data gained from a much larger sample size, or it may be designed for the purposes of gathering nutritional, epidemiological or other information not normally encompassed within anthropology.

## References

Hubert A. (1990) Applying anthropology to the epidemiology of cancer, *Anthropology Today*, 5: 7–11.

Hubert, A., Jeannel, D., Tuppin, P. and Thé, G.de (1992) Anthropology and epidemiology: a pluridisciplinary approach to nasopharyngeal carcinoma. In Tursz, T., Pagano, J.S., Ablachi, D.V., Thé, G.de, Lenoir, G. and Pearson, G.R. (eds) *Epstein-Barr Virus and Associated Diseases,* INSERM and John Libbe Eurotext: 775–788.

Macbeth, H., Collinson, P. and Collingwood Bakeo, A. (2002) Changes in beer-drinking and pub-going habits in U.K.: indications from a small Oxfordshire study in 2001, *Alimenta Populorum*, 2(1): 11–21.

Mead, M. (1945) *Manual for the Study of Food Habits*, National Academy of Science, Washington D.C. 84.

# APPENDIX

## INTERVIEW GUIDE

What follows is a guide to topics which can be used in semi-directed discussions in each household or family group; interviews should preferably be carried out with members of each generation. Specific codings may be used to indicate generation and/or any other appropriate attribute, within the general coding for that family group.

### Identification of the family:
Name
Members of the household
Place of residence

### Type of housing

### Daily life
Household organisation and schedule
Who is in charge of food shopping?
Who cooks?
Household cleaning, etc.
Meals taken at home (who eats?, when?, where?)
Meals taken out of home (who eats?, when?, where?)

### Food and shopping:
*According to type of products*
Market
Supermarket
Specialty shops
Grocery
Delicatessen
Others
Time spent for shopping and frequency
Distance covered
Is a shopping list used?

*Motivation for choices*
Family habit
Children's demands
Publicity (TV commercials, magazines, radio, posters, etc.; ask examples)
Price
Quality
Quantity
Other

*Domestic production: today and in the past*
Vegetable garden, orchard, chickens, etc.
What?
Since when?
Who is in charge?
When started or stopped, and for what reasons?
Gifts and exchanges with the family members or neighbours or friends
– for direct consumption, preserving or sale?
Gathering wild plants, hunting and fishing
Produce collected
– for direct consumption, preserving or sale?

**How shopping was done before the advent of large-scale distribution (super-markets, etc.), by the preceding generation or during elderly informants' youth**
*Household preserves*
Types of product
Where does one get them?
Types of preserves (freezing, sterilising, jams, pickles, etc.)
Estimation of quantities
Freezing
Freezer or not in the house
Types of frozen food: own production, bought,
Estimation of frequency of consumption
Other means of keeping food: cellar, etc.
How was food preserving carried out before supermarkets
– e.g. by preceding generation or during youth of elderly informants

**Food consumption : utensils, techniques and products given here should be adapted to the country of study**
How is cooking organised?
Who prepares the meals?
Who decides the menus?
When is meal composition decided: by week, some days before, at the time of preparing the meal ?
Time and period of day spent cooking (morning, evening, weekends)

*Kitchen equipment*
cooker, ovens ( microwave, etc.), gas, electricity
Mixers, and other electric equipment
Types of pots and pans

*Cooking techniques*
Preferred techniques and their frequency
Seasonal differences
Steaming

Stews
Boiled
Baked
Grilled
Fried
Raw

*Learning how to cook*
Where does one learn the recipes from?
Cookbooks? which? where obtained? used when ?

*Types of dishes*
Soups
Stews
Baked dishes and casseroles
Grilled and barbecued
Fried
Salads
Others ( according to local cuisines)
Give recipes of regularly recurring dishes
Are dishes different according to season ?

*Spices and condiments*
Spicy food, use of herbs and spices most used
Preferred tastes of the person interviewed and his/her close family

*Fats*
Types of oil (olive, peanut, soy, safflower, etc.) frequency of use and types used,
preferences
Margarine (which kind)
Butter
Pork fat (drippings)
Cream

*'sauces' and condiments added to a meal (put on the table)*
Mayonnaise,
Salad cream, bottled sauces, etc.
Tomato sauce
Garlic sauce, etc.
Which are most frequently used?

**Products consumed by the household:**
Specify the different kinds and estimate how much and how often

*Meats, fish and eggs*
Meats (list according to local traditions)
Fish (list...)
Shellfish, etc.
Hams and delicatessen
Eggs

*Vegetables*
Greens (list...)
Other 'fruit' vegetables (tomatoes, aubergine, peppers, etc. – list...)
Roots and tubers

*Cereals (types of bread, pasta, breakfast, rice) whole or refined*

*Milk and milk products*
Milk (whole, half fat, low calorie, plus vitamins, etc.)
Yoghurt
Butter
Cream
Cheeses (list...)

*fruit* (list...)
Dried fruits
Fresh fruit
Frozen fruit

*Other*
Beans and pulses
Pastries and sweets (home made or bought)
Other specialties

Preferred products and/or most often consumed
Why?
Products rarely consumed
Why?
Products never consumed
Why?

What are the dishes, drinks or foods that you do not eat but your parents ate
or eat?
Why?

What are the dishes, drinks, foods that you eat but your parents do not eat or
ate?
Why?

**Daily meals**
Composition and times
Breakfast
Lunch
Tea or snacks (when?, what kind?)
Dinner
Meals eaten outside home
Who and where?
Composition
Snacks: who and what kind?
What is thought of as essential in a meal (without it would not be a meal)?
Table setting and decoration
Who serves, who is served first?
Who gets favourite treatment at table (special diet, dishes, best bits, etc.)?
Conversation or not, about what
TV or radio during meals?
Which is the most important meal of the day: for what reasons?
Differences in the organisation of the meal in the preceding generation (or the following)?
Give the menu of a feast, or special occasion, with the drinks. Christmas or New Year (adapt for the country/the society/the culture)

*Drinks*
What is drunk during meals?
If wine/beer (etc.), what kind? from where?
How much is drunk by whom?
Do you have a cellar?
Is wine/beer (etc.) drunk mainly at home or where?
Other alcoholic drinks: sherry, port, cocktails, etc.
Drunk by whom and how much?
Drinks on special occasions
Drinks outside meals: tea, coffee, sodas, beer, etc.
Drunk by whom and how much?
Mineral water
What kind?

*Interesting comparisons*
Are there differences in drinking patterns and products between generations?
Remarks on the food ways of the in-laws (and tastes of the spouse)
Important changes in lifestyle between generations and consequences on food habits today. What are the new foods which have become usual?

**What is a healthy diet**
Is it different from a tasty or gourmet diet?
Any special diets (slimming, diabetes, etc. for what reasons? for whom?)

Is beauty linked to diet?
When you look at someone, what aspect of the body makes you think they are in good health ?
Give the menu of an ideal meal (without restriction of budget)

**Household composition** (could be done at the start of interview):
Head of the family (male or female)
Date and place of birth
Preceding places of residence
Residence today
Education
Occupation
Family situation and number of children

# 4. 'TELL ME WHAT YOU EAT AND YOU WILL TELL ME WHO YOU ARE'

## METHODOLOGICAL NOTES ON THE INTERACTION BETWEEN RESEARCHER AND INFORMANTS IN THE ANTHROPOLOGY OF FOOD

*F. Xavier Medina*

## Introduction

This chapter concerns the interaction between researcher and informant in relation to the study of the anthropology of food. The relationship between researchers and informants is one of the main tools on which anthropologists rely in order to gain an insight into unknown facts. Information obtained (and later processed) by researchers through interviews, is a crucial asset for the sociocultural study of human food habits. However, information, based solely on informants' assertions, is subject to certain constraints and biases. Exactly which ones depends on the kind of material the researcher hopes to gain. These restrictions may be removed or at least reduced using other qualitative techniques such as the researcher's participant observation.

What follows is an attempt to approach some of these issues by reflecting on some of the tools most used in social anthropology to gain information. More specifically, I discuss the nature of fieldwork; I stress that the structure of interviews turns on informants' construction of discourse through the process of interacting with a researcher. I conclude with some reflections on the role of participant observation.

## Researchers and Informants

As Margaret Mead explains in the account of her Samoan fieldwork experience, the only instructions her teacher, Franz Boas, gave her were that she had to be prepared to apparently waste time, since all an anthropologist could do was to listen to her informants (Mead 1972). Boas' advice lies within a methodological context associated with a particular style of interaction between informants and researchers. The intention of researchers is to gain a clear knowledge of situations, about which, at first, they know nothing and to which they have access through very few links. One of these links, perhaps the most important, is an informant, i.e. a person who is part of the society being studied and who knows its norms and values because he or she was socialised within it.

The style of interaction between a researcher and the people he or she works with is obviously crucial for the development of the analysis. Getting closer to somebody demands a more or less fluid feedback on both sides and a certain degree of 'trust', which may be dialectic (as occurs in an interview), or factive (as occurs when anthropologists actively try to participate in the lives of the people they are observing).

## Open Interviews to Obtain Information

The style of one's research will vary according to one's approach and goals. For example, in my own research on the construction of ethnicity by Basque migrants to Catalonia via food habits (Medina 2000), I chose to analyse informants' discourse, using material I had gained through open, semi-directed interviews. This analysis allowed me to investigate the construction of ethnicity from within, i.e. how the members of the specific group constructed it for themselves.

In this particular case, therefore, paying attention to informants' discourse was of prime importance since the discourse was itself a social act, informing us about the processes and interests involved in the construction of their ethnicity. Food is, without doubt, an outstanding element in this sort of construction. Food is used for self-recognition as well as for differentiating oneself from others. In this respect, the discourses themselves were as interesting as the food practices, because it was the elaboration of the social construction, rather than of the reality itself, that was the objective of this particular research.

I believe that the only way of approaching this sort of topic is by considering the construction carried out *from within*, by taking into account what is regarded as relevant by the very people who participate in this process. For this reason, the most useful method involved semi-directed open interviews, which respected the informants' agency while still directing the research according to the researcher's pre-planned aims and interests.

Interviews provide researchers with various methodological advantages. Firstly, a direct, face-to-face relationship with an informant favours the creation of a certain complicity and reliance that may break pre-existing barriers. Secondly, the researcher may pose questions and change them along the way, stressing one or another aspect, if the answer is not 'satisfactory' or if contradictory responses occur. A question may even be reformulated differently during further interviews. A third, important factor (as noted above) is that, as opposed to what happens with questionnaires, the researcher may count not only on learning the intellectual points made by informants, but on hearing examples based on direct experience as well, while all the time observing the respondent. These factors may play a crucial role in being able to elaborate on particular points at the time or later and to put them into their appropriate contexts.

The use of open interviews, even though they are partially guided, provides a useful range of information. There is no doubt that the freedom of expression enjoyed by an informant makes his or her discourse, and consequently the analysis, richer and more varied. Because of this, the ability of both parties to relax and get to know one another a bit better often leads to fuller answers and a rich store of illuminating examples. As Scheuch (1973) argues, the main advantage of the interview is its flexibility, i.e. the high degree of procedural adaptation to each interviewee and to each situation. As a result, the more familiar communicative context during an in-depth interview and the often higher rapport generate more complete answers and quite rich anecdotal material.

These examples, which may sometimes seem superfluous, constitute a corpus of information, which can provide a researcher with a great deal of important data. These data are potentially useful for future investigations for two reasons: (1) they answer directly the questions posed to informants, and (2) they indirectly give information about issues, which were not envisaged at the beginning and only appear later on. Also and very importantly, such a corpus of information provides a wider framework, on which a researcher may rely in order to contrast an interviewee's statements with other data and observations. For example, a statement, regarded as dubious by the researcher, whether the interviewee intended to mislead or not, may be compared, and at times even corrected, with the help of other more indirect material, such as information given by the same or other interviewees (see also González and Mataix this volume).

Informants' discourse is, of course, a highly selective, mediated portrayal of reality, which has to be interpreted by the researcher. In this sense, as García (1996) argues, discourse is not just a vehicle of information, but must be regarded as an object of study itself, to be observed and analysed. Similarly, as Gondar (1995) observes in his article on anorexia as a food disorder, it is important to bear in mind that informants, apart from being the source of a story, are themselves historians. This is because they are at the same time creators and narrators of their accounts, even though their storytelling may well be more narrative than analytical. Thus, informants are not only 'texts' but authors as well, and they must be observed and treated as such.

## The Researcher–Informant Relationship: Interactions and Possible Clashes

As with any other social relationship, the bond between researchers and informants has its own conventions and reciprocal interests. Inevitably, it involves constant negotiations between the two interlocutors. The meeting, which is planned from the start as a vehicle for obtaining information, directly benefits the researcher whereas the informant, whose presence is apparently voluntary and altruistic, does not seem to gain anything. Interaction of this kind, which is constructed in terms of this initial 'inequality', may suffer from occasional 'clashes'. These should be understood as a failure by the researcher to explain adequately his or her specific needs and interests and the usefulness and aim of the research itself.

The Austrian social anthropologists, Kutalek (2000) and Heidenreich (2000), have, each on the basis of their own fieldwork, pinpointed some interesting aspects of the interaction between researcher and informant. Both anthropologists used in the titles of their respective articles highly significant statements. The title of Kutalek's article begins: 'They will tell you only what they believe you want to hear'. In fact, as in any interaction between individuals, there is a manifest multiplicity of intentions on the part of both partners. There is also a series of 'introductions of the person' or of each 'I' interviewed to the other interlocutor. It is important to remember that interviewees introduce themselves to the researcher both individually and collectively as members of the group they belong to. For all these reasons, informants tend to provide carefully selected aspects of reality. This is partly because they wish to offer the best possible image, exposing those aspects which are generally believed to be the most valued. It is also partly because informants may develop their own interpretation of what the researcher is seeking and, thus make a subjective selection of those aspects of reality which they believe to be useful, while omitting others which they regard as less relevant. It is furthermore possible that informants may simply not mention a number of factors which they consider to be self-evident but which are not at all obvious to the researcher.

The following example is taken from my own fieldwork about Basque migrants in Catalonia. Various informants who were asked about the dishes they prepared and consumed daily in their homes and with their families, gave answers which almost exclusively concerned typical Basque cooking. They neglected to mention any other kind of cooking practices, assuming that I was not interested in that kind of information. Only at my insistence and after further specific questions, most of which arose from participant observation in the informants' homes, did I obtain information which was more detailed and closer to the reality of these people's daily consumption. Given that in this research I was focusing on the informants' ethnic discourses, the answers *per se* were an invaluable source of data and of reflection. Yet, it is worth noting that the information obtained was, in itself, clearly biased and misleading as a possible source of information on the daily food consumption and 'real' cooking practices of the informants.

A rather different case is exemplified by the opening sentence of Heidenreich's (2000) article, 'If I tell you so, I may be lying'. Here, the context is very different from that of Kutalek and its implications take us way beyond the mere involuntary bias, into a conscious and deceitful distortion of information by local interlocutors. Almost by definition, researchers intrude upon some of the more intimate corners of informants' lives. This intrusion may take the form of broaching issues which informants find hard to talk about for various reasons, such as personal shyness, embarrassment or, as mentioned above, the wish to give as positive an image as possible. Other reasons may be the lack of interest or belief in the usefulness of the researcher's task, the wish for the interview to be over as quickly as possible or, simply, the refusal to reveal specific information to somebody alien to the group. In all these cases the kind of information offered may be deliberately wrong.

A significant example here is that of the informant, who worked at a mid-management level in business and who asserted that she always bought the best food and never spared any expense when it came to her family's meals. She said she always used fresh and top-quality foodstuffs and never resorted to frozen and ready-cooked dishes even though this meant extra time devoted to shopping and cooking:

.... always fresh. If I cook fish it will be cod, and fresh!... This frozen stuff, pizzas and croquettes... I prepare them myself... God knows what's in ready-made food.

However, a glimpse at her kitchen cupboards and freezer revealed a rather different story, for there were both frozen and tinned ready-cooked foods, etc. of various sorts. My surprise led me to ask her husband – also my informant – a direct question at a time when the woman was out of the house. The man revealed that he was responsible for the presence of such ready-cooked foodstuffs because he, in practice, was the one who did the shopping and the cooking most days. In fact, his wife's schedule did not allow her to carry out such activities during the week. The woman only did the cooking occasionally and mainly at the weekend, whereas the husband was in charge of his wife's and his two children's meals most of the time. From Mondays to Fridays she usually ate lunch out, as did her husband, while during the day the children were left in the charge of their grandparents. In the evening, when the woman came home from work, she found dinner ready since her husband arrived back much earlier than she did.

In this case, the informant's statement at the time of the interview was only partially correct. She does value fresh products and traditional cooking, and her discourse clearly conveys such values. Yet it does not say anything about the food practices in her home and how they related to her family. The omission of the fact that she is not the one who usually cooks, which was later on confirmed through participant observation, tells us a great deal about the image that this informant wished to offer the researcher. Not doing the shopping and the cooking herself, and using ready-cooked, frozen or industrially prepared products were perceived by her as facts that might offer a negative image of the way she cared for members of her family who, according to her, deserved 'the best'. The link between food and health becomes obvious here. One cannot 'play with health', as the Spanish say. Thus, the concealment of information on the part of the interviewee was, on this occasion, deliberate and motivated by interests which strictly concerned the researcher-informant relationship.

Lastly, and closely related to what has been shown so far, one cannot lose sight of the fact that there is a gap between subjects' discourse and their actual practices. Discursive logic is frequently constructed around ideas which often do not necessarily come from the food habits themselves, but from sociocultural conventions conveyed by discourses which are very diverse in their origin (traditional, medical, commercial, etc.). As Gracia (1996) argues, the meaning of everyday food issues is complex, and the various factors which define them (e.g. ethics, identity and hierarchy) become symbolic elements which may increase any gap between discussants. For this reason researchers must never forget that informants' discourses are always expressed through the sociocultural sieve of their own ideology and scale of values.

Gracia (1996) gives as an example of this gap the organisation of the familial food budget. According to him food money is a priority within the household budget, since it ensures the group's physical survival. Other expenses are sorted out only afterwards. However, as he goes on to demonstrate, this may not be what happens in practice, even though such is the way that things are perceived by the informants. Food money, in fact, turns out to be the most flexible item of household budgets, while priority is given to other expenses such as the mortgage, taxes, etc., which are more difficult to modify. Despite this, and under direct questioning, informants usually mention food expenses as the most important and the least changeable item in their budgets. This is due to a genuine perception of food expenses as a priority, and not to a deliberate wish to alter information given to the researcher. Nevertheless, the gap between discourse and reality does exist.

In this sense, as García (1996) argues, informants' discourse, as well as the informants themselves and their reactions during the interviews, must be observed and analysed in their own context. On the one hand, one must pay attention to informants' reactions, possible doubts and reluctance to answer questions. Heidenreich (2000: 17) wrote 'I found that these reactions to my inquiries contained much more information than simple and direct answers'. On the other hand, one must consider an interviewee's personal and 'material' context. For this reason it is advisable to hold the interviews in environments, which are strongly associated with the interviewees and the topic, e.g. in their kitchen or pantry, where they are surrounded by personal and everyday items. Such items may provide a researcher with interesting complementary information and also a starting point for the formulation of new questions.

## Participant Observation

Already by the beginning of the 1980s, Garine (1980) had drawn attention to the need to combine and use various sources of information rationally, and he put special emphasis on qualitative approaches. These kinds of techniques, especially participant observation, make it possible to obtain a great breadth of information, which allows us to correct biases which may be present in interlocutors' discourses. As explained above, these biases are always part of an informants' subjectivity, which, of course interacts with the also inevitable subjectivity of the researcher. Such unavoidable interaction between the two interlocutors is a characteristic of which the anthropologist must always be aware. It is a factor to be taken into account whenever carrying out fieldwork, interpreting data and elaborating the final text. It is from this very perspective that one might be able to bridge the gap between reality and information which is consciously or unconsciously given in a partial or erroneous way inherent to the informants' discourse.

One of the most useful instruments for this purpose is precisely that of participant observation, where the researcher spends a considerable, continuous period of time living intensively with those being studied, learning small nuances in their language and, through participation in all activities, gaining a deeper understanding of those activities and their social context. It is a technique, which places the interaction between researcher and investigated subjects within a wider context, as it goes beyond the verbal register. This wider context includes a multiplicity of aspects which, because shared by anthropologists and informants at the same level, considerably increase the breadth of the researcher's understanding. Thus, participant observation is a research method which allows one to pay more attention to informants' views, because anthropologists try to become part of what is being observed while keeping an ethnographic distance in order to analyse critically the various situations and the oral information about them.

The difficult construction of the relationship between researcher and informant, who are in the ultimate analysis interlocutors at the same level, establishes an interaction which is always dynamic and different in each case. Yet these interviewing techniques are ideally complemented by participant observation, if we are to acknowledge adequately the informants' perspective. This technique of combining interviewing with participant observation allows researchers to interpret and analyse informants' discourse with a better knowledge of facts. It enables clearer perspectives and a broader range of information. Above all it takes into consideration the subjects' own points of view.

# References

García, J.L. (1996) El análisis del discurso en la antropología social. In García, J.L. (ed.) *Etnolingüística y análisis del discurso*, Instituto Aragonés de Antropología/del Estado Español, Zaragoza: 11–17.

Garine, I. de (1980) Une anthropologie alimentaire des français? *Ethnologie Française*, X(3), 227–238.

Gondar, M. (1995) O exótico como ponte cultural. As claves d'un simposio. In *Anorexia: Dieta, Estética, Crenzas*, Sección de Etnomedicina, Museo do Pobo Galego, Santiago de Compostela: 9–21.

Gracia, M. (1996) El decalage entre el discurso del informante y sus prácticas: el caso de la alimentación. In García, J.L. (ed.) *Etnolingüística y análisis del discurso*, Instituto Aragonés de Antropología/Federación de Asociaciones de Antropología del Estado Español, Zaragoza: 65–84.

Heidenreich, F. (2000) If I told you this, I would be lying. On the difficulty of obtaining answers in ethnomedical field research: reflections on aspects of my fieldwork with a Seereer healer in the Republic of Senegal, *Viennese Ethnomedicine Newsletter*, II(3): 16–20.

Kutalek, R. (2000) They will only tell you what they believe you want to hear. Reactions to my research on traditional medicine in Tanzania, *Viennese Ethnomedicine Newsletter*, II(3): 3–16.

Mead, M. (1972) *Blackberry Winter: my earlier years*, William Morrow, New York.

Medina, F.X. (2000) *Vascos en Barcelona: una aproximación al estudio de la etnicidad desde la antropología*, Universitat de Barcelona, Barcelona. (unpublished PhD thesis).

Scheuch, E.K. (1973) La entrevista en la investigación social. In König, R. (ed.) *Tratado de Sociología Empírica*, volume 1, Tecnos, Madrid: 166–230.

# 5. FOOD, IDENTITY, IDENTIFICATION

*Jeremy MacClancy*

**A**nthropologists need to be very cautious when talking about 'identity'. For several reasons.

Firstly, 'identity' is such a catch-all term that almost anything can come within its compass. A seemingly empty vessel fillable with almost any content, it can be used as a general framing device for a surprising range of ethnographic data. Some might think this a strength of the term, its versatility and possible extension being of potential benefit to social anthropology. After all, they might argue, key concepts are always inherently vague. The trouble is, adopting this style may well lead to us anthropologists imposing *our* notion of identity upon unmarked aspects of others' cultures. The danger is that we may extol or assiduously analyse a part of others' lives, which they themselves regard either as of little importance, or as not just restricted to themselves but common to many. We start to find symbols where none at present exists. Perilous procedure this, for the resulting ethnography may tell us more about the imaginative power, the classificatory ingenuity of its author, than about the way the people studied regard themselves. And who, may I ask, is more interested in studying anthropologists themselves than in studying what they have to say?

Secondly 'identity', as an abstract noun, may well make some think of an entity with clear boundaries to be traced and sharp contours to be defined. It may well make some think of an entity fixed in time or coasting through it, impervious to vicissitudes. Yet it was Fredrik Barth (1969) who argued over thirty years ago that identity is essentially relational: that to study an identity, one must look at what it is defined against, and how that definition may change over time. Thirdly, as a noun, it may appear to some as agent-less, autonomous and sufficient unto itself, as though benefiting from a preordained independence. This does not square with the ethnographic record (see, e.g. Eriksen 1993). Fourthly, as an abstract noun, it tends often to be used in the singular, as though plural identities were the exception, not the commonplace that they here are. Among other commentators, MacClancy (1996) has underlined the fallacy of this misuse. Fifthly, 'identity' is usually regarded as an unproblematic category, rather than as one fragmented in nature and constantly challenged. MacClancy (1997) exposed just how untenable that position is in the contemporary world.

For all these sorts of reasons and in these contexts, 'identity' is a very tricky concept for anthropologists to employ. It appears to be an unjustifiably arbitrary manner of delineating others' lives in academic terms. An oversimplifier of complex realities, its use runs the risk of turning the abstract into the substantial, of sculpting a shape out of the almost formless, and of playing fast and loose with the temporal dimension. Of course this does not mean we should not study how others deploy the concept. Far from it. Being aware of these potential pitfalls *should* make us more sensitive to the ways others use the term.

Perhaps then, it is best for anthropologists to study others' exploitation of ideas about identity but to talk among themselves of 'modes of identification'. The change is not merely semantic. It has numerous advantages. First, it shifts attention from the static to the dynamic, from focusing on a particular point in time to watching the evolutions of the processual. Second, it takes us from an overconcern with the singular to a challenging emphasis on the plural: I say *challenging*, because it forces those who wish to claim a solitary mode of identification to argue their case, to persuade us why they think there is only one such mechanism operating within their research area. Third, its use pushes aside a pseudoautonomous 'identity' for the sake of reintroducing, in a fully integrated manner, the roles, motivations and actions of agents in any identificatory process. On this account 'identities' do not simply exist, as though floating independently through the ether; rather individuals or groups initiate or perform actions in particular contexts for identificatory purposes. Fourth, by making us observe how the locals shift and swerve, trying to negotiate the deployment of these modes, study of them helps us overcome the above worries about imposing categories on others. For what we would be doing here is not foisting categories of our own device on the locals, but observing the ways they use their own categories, to what end, to what effect. Here we would be tracing the means employed by others to isolate an identifiable identity within the global flows of today, which otherwise threaten to carry all with them. I recognise that it is easier to conduct this kind of research in areas where local notions of 'identity' have become deeply politicised than in places where political conflict has not taken quite that form.

## Modes of Identification

Modes of identification are many and operate at many different levels. The scheme I here present is only to be taken as illustrative or suggestive. It is intended as a springboard for thought, not as a prescription etched in acid. In the same vein, I should add that the particular modes catalogued below are not to be seen as mutually exclusive *taxa*, as a series of separate pigeon-holes for packets of knowledge. Rather, they should be viewed as a loose collection of overlapping themes, with the reader well aware of their provisional nature and expository purpose. In other words, if our aims were slightly different, no doubt so would be the modes isolated.

## The Literary Mode of Identification, or What to Read, How?

For me, the key source of information here is newspapers, which are, most surprisingly, a still deeply neglected fount of data for anthropologists. The range and sorts of relevant information here is very broad. For instance:

a)   reviews of restaurants
b)   interviews with chefs
c)   letters to the editor
d)   editorials
e)   articles by columnists
f)   feature articles
g)   news on certain kinds of events: the staging of competitions, the giving of prizes, the presence of politicians at key food-based events, etc.

In the course of my own research on local notions of cuisine in the general Basque area of northern Spain, I have encountered much material of great interest in pieces from all of these six categories. Of course, I have often had to read 'against the grain', scanning articles or letters which are not directly concerned with food matters but which may well still contain highly appropriate material: the gems, we might call them, hidden within the coal. It pays to read fast and to learn how to skim; and the more one comes close to commanding a body of knowledge the faster one can skim.

Next in our survey come books and, again, relevant ones may be of an exceptionally wide variety:

(a)   cookbooks: both essential and potentially profoundly misleading. Above all, a cookbook should not be taken as indicative of what locals ate in the time and area it was written. Books, even cookbooks, are written for a diversity of reasons and it is often more profitable to enquire *why* they have been written than to analyse their contents in an uncritical manner. Also, cookbooks are literary products and have to be seen as such. It was Evelyn Waugh, after all, who said his favourite bedtime reading was the books of Elizabeth David.

All cookbooks have fictional dimensions. The question is: of what kind and to what degree? Some, for instance, act as deeply idealised folkloric records; the authors of these salvage ethnographies are concerned to 'save' seemingly traditional recipes before they are lost. Other books are lengthy expressions of cultural nostalgia (Fragner 2000). The script here seems to be: 'this is the world we have already lost, but which we can try to re-create through cooking'. The world they have lost, however, is almost always rural, green and harmonious; there are no ugly towns, dirty chimney stacks or working-class discontent in the visions they perpetuate. Cookbooks may also appeal to the aspirations of their readers, feeding their fantasies about the identities they wish to achieve rather than lending substance to the identities they already possess. Thus contemporary cookbooks which focus on the folkloric, the nostalgic, or the aspirational (as so many do) may tell us less about culinary conditions than about collective imaginations, present-day values, and popular dreams, hopes and aims. They have to be seen not as descriptive documents but as prescriptive ones, giving us an inkling of the culinary worlds their authors would like to see.

It is important here to remember that the claims to existence of any contemporary nation are partly legitimated by its self-vaunted possession of a prestigious culture, and that an ideologically significant part of a culture may well be its distinctive cuisine. For these reasons, the modern rise of nationalism and regionalism has boosted the production of cookbooks. Indeed in some cases it may well be the nationalists or regionalists themselves who are funding the publication of these books. It is common for claims to be made about the great age of much local cuisine. For, as Zubaida (2000: 41) argues, 'This supposed historical antiquity and continuity are cited as, somehow, a confirmation of the authenticity and superiority of the present-day national cuisine. History, then, becomes the measure of national virtue, including food.' According to this line, eating in a local manner is to consume history, to uphold virtue.

When looking at a Basque cookbook for the first time, the questions I usually ask myself are: Who wrote this? For whom? When? Where? What position did the author hold? What local contexts can this book be fitted into? Who are the publishers? Who funded this book? What might the author have gained from producing it? What interests, beyond the immediately individual, was he or she seeking to promote? How successful was the book? What image of the Basqueland, of local society, and of local cooking is the author trying to portray? What are the proportions between the different kinds of dishes (meat, fish, vegetable, sweet, etc.)? Are significant proportions of the dishes from distinct sub-zones of the area in question? In other words, these books are not simply to be broached, but to be interrogated.

(b) Novels, especially bad novels: the less artistry the local author displays the better, for then all the more likely he or she is to tell us about local life in a relatively unmediated, unpolished manner. From reading local novels, I have been able to learn about, for example, the social importance granted to cultivating a fine palate, the role of food in romance, and the centrality of feasting.

(c) <u>Memoirs</u>: another neglected source of data, most likely because the trawl, on occasion, can be long and the catch relatively meagre. However in my Basque case, the sorts of information I have been able to glean from examples of this genre include accounts of recently defunct rules of behaviour and forms of interaction, both formal and informal, as well as eulogies to the local diet and styles of cooking. As in other domains of activity, what is more important here is often the mode of praise rather than its content.

## The Ritual Mode of Identification, or What Events to Observe; How?

The rituals investigated may vary enormously in scope, from the intensely local to the national. They may range from a small, communal meal eaten collectively by all the members of a hamlet during its annual fiesta to a particular day in the calendar associated regionally or nationally with certain foods, e.g. the inclusion of elvers (now a very expensive dish) in Christmas Eve dinner, the main Yuletide feast in the Basqueland. I remember attending the annual fiesta of a small village in the Central Zone of the autonomous province of Navarre, northern Spain, where the *dia del pueblo* ('day of the village') was not only celebrated by a collective meal but by the cooking, in the central square, of the main course in an extraordinarily large flat cooking dish. As some locals told me with pride, it had belonged to the refectory of a former seminary within the village. They were not just concelebrating community by eating together but having the communal meal cooked on an instrumental product of their common history.

Also, events here may be defined in terms of occupation or leisure-group (e.g. the gastronomic societies of the Basque area), or of the stages within the annual agricultural cycle [e.g. in the Basqueland, the ritual opening of the first cider barrel or the first bottles of *txakoli* (a local, somewhat acidic white wine) of the new harvest].

## The Historiographic Mode of Identification, or Whose Past to Study?

This mode is particularly pockmarked by difficulties. Thanks to the work of academics such as Hobsbawm and Ranger (1983) and Boissevain (1992), it is now extremely well-established that many so-called traditions are in fact relatively modern inventions or recent revitalisations of almost moribund customs. And that the reasons why people today maintain particular traditions, cloaking them in the trappings of the past, may be very different from why they or their predecessors maintained them in previous decades.

This is especially so when we come to questions of identity, for it appears that the upholders or promoters of an identity often feel it necessary to supply that identity with a past, even if much of that past was specially created for the purpose. This is very much a question of the production of particular pasts for the present. Nostalgia can here play an eminently practical role, as the praise of a particular view of the past while keeping one eye on a particular, wished-for view of the future.

For instance, in my own research on the creation and evolution of gastronomic societies in the Basque area, I was very conscious throughout that I had to constantly sift the seemingly historical material which so many local eulogisers used when speaking about this regionally distinctive institution. A particular image of these societies, it appeared, was so useful to particular sectors within Basque nationalism that most of the popular conceptions about the societies are best regarded as more mythical than factual. Many nationalist writers, it appeared, wanted it believed that the societies were the traditional homes of a democratic egalitarianism where, in a playful inversion of the normal order, men acted as the chefs. I found that much of that statement can be radically questioned (MacClancy, n.d.).

## The Culinary Mode of Identification, or What do Cooks do? How? For What Reasons?

This could just as easily be called the 'careerist' or 'self-promotional' mode of identification, for here I wish to draw attention to the ways chefs can advance their own standing by publicising a certain kind of cuisine. It is relatively easy for a loosely associated group of chefs to promote a relatively new cuisine, especially if they claim to be its best, original and most innovative practitioners. This is relevant to our purposes as, in areas where cooking is already highly valued and local identity strongly stressed, the local chefs may well phrase their cuisine in localist terms. By the simultaneous promotion of both their food and the area, they win the support of local journalists, eager for easy copy, and of regionalist politicians, keen to find further ways to boost regional distinctiveness and pride.

The main example I think of here is the creation of the 'New Basque Cuisine' by a huddle of Basque chefs in the 1980s, who adapted the innovations of the French *nouvelle cuisine* to the local context. Legitimating their pretensions by the national laudits and prizes some of them won, they furthered their aims by granting seemingly endless interviews to local and national journalists and by being ever ready to pose with politicians at appropriate gastronomic events. Some of the politicians returned the favour by making them the latest winners of prizes dedicated to successful practitioners of regional culture. It is easy, and not overcynical, to ask how much of this would have happened if the chefs had called their cooking by another term: e.g. 'the New Cuisine of San Sebastián' (the city where almost all of them worked)?

## The Local Mode of Identification, or Who are 'We'? Who are 'They'?

Much of this could also be included in the ritual mode of identification. Local modes include:

a)   local cultivation of crops;
b)   local ways of cultivating crops;
c)   the cultivation of certain crops, valued and praised by locals;
d)   foraged food, locally collected, acclaimed by locals;
e)   local terms for foods and toponyms;
f)   traditional festivities;
g)   the discourse of food.

In the village where I am usually based when conducting my Basque-area research, my landlords (with whom I ate every day) liked to boast of how much of what we were eating had been produced by their own hand, on their own land. They tended to underline how much better it tasted than much shop-bought produce. My landlord's father would stress how delicious were the particular strains of fruit or salad vegetable they had chosen to cultivate. They and other villagers underlined how creamy the local milk was and how distinctive its flavour. My landlords, like other locals, would also praise certain foods from certain villages, e.g. the kidney beans of Genevilla, a village twenty kilometres to the west, as being especially good.

They may take patent pride when presenting a certain local product (e.g. the village's wine, its olive oil), emphasising how 'natural' it is, i.e. how relatively free from chemical additives. One September evening, as the harvested grapes were being ditched into collection vats, one worker siphoned off some fresh grape juice for me. 'Try that,' he said, '100 percent pure! And you can't say that about what's sold in the shops! Full of chemicals that stuff!' On Sunday evenings, I usually ate with my landlord who often took delight in showing me how well he knew the countryside by cooking us a meal centred around the undomesticated products he had foraged that afternoon from spots in the sur-rounding countryside (whose location he would never tell me): wild asparagus, mushrooms, crayfish, etc., washed down with the village wine and 'mountain tea' (an infusion made of a local herb I could not identify).

My landlords took pleasure in pointing out to me how even the local terms for a few fruits (such as apricots) were different in their village and those immediately around it from the terms used in the next valley. Several locals were also greatly concerned that all the toponyms within the municipal bound-aries be catalogued and so saved for posterity. They were rightly worried that with the rejection of agriculture as an occupation by most of the village youth and the recent *concentración parcelaria* (reorganisation of all the arable land within the municipality into larger fields, which could be more efficiently worked), most toponyms would fall into disuse and be forgotten. To them, these verbal markers of their agricultural space were too valuable a local heritage to

*Figure 5.1*   Food as part of local identity: the weekly dinner of an age-set, in their clubhouse, in a Navarran village

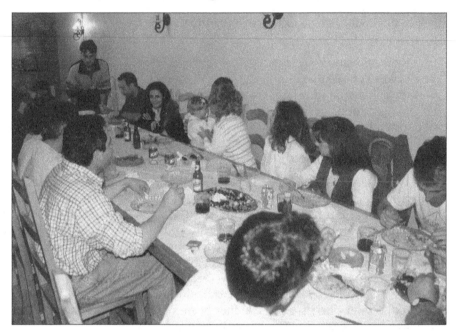

be lost so easily. So they raised some of the money to have the task carried out professionally, and did what remained themselves.

Traditional festivities included the weekly dinners of some age-sets within the village. One form of village classification is the division of everyone into age-sets, each covering about a five-year period. If the members of an age-set are active and enthusiastic, they buy a small house or storage building, and convert it into their own premises. Its main purpose is for the holding of dinners every Saturday night and every night during the week-long annual fiestas of the village. A different pair of members prepares the meal each time, and clears up afterwards. If successful, these meals can be lengthy, lively and loud, with well-charged members singing, debating, and not moving onto the bars of the village until one or two in the morning.

At both meals with my landlords and with the age-set I was attached to, it was important to note: what was being eaten, in what terms was it being assessed, and how was it judged? Information collected in this way may provide insights into the way food is locally valued, while the degree of criticism, its fineness, and how publicly it may be stated are all indicators of how concerned locals are about the quality of what they eat. They are also indicators of the extent to which locals recognise a refined palate and the ability to talk about it as a hallmark of savoir-faire, as a necessary skill for those who wish to be regarded even minimally civilised, or as a sure sign of snobbery. For what a Navarran smallholder might regard as a perfectly reasonable comment on his wife's cooking and which would be accepted by her as such (e.g. 'Good but a little overcooked and too much salt. We really shouldn't buy so much frozen fish; best to keep to fresh when we can afford it.'), his English counterpart might judge as verging on the insulting, and pretentious to boot, while traditionalist members of the English upper class might view any such concern with the quality of the food and the desire to speak about it at length as an index of poor upbringing: 'Always vulgar to talk about the food, my dear'.

## Fieldwork, Participant Observation and Other Intellectual Excursions

Other social anthropologists contributing to this volume have already discussed some of the pros and cons of fieldwork and participant observation (e.g. Hubert, Medina). I wish here only to underscore those points my colleagues have not themselves stressed.

My first point has to be that much of what I learnt about food habits while in the village, I learnt because I was living there for an extended period (just under two years), have kept on going back at least annually, and have consistently tried as much as possible to participate in the tasks of the community: especially assisting both my smallholder landlord (pruning vines, harvesting grapes, 'milking' [to use the local term] olive trees, stacking bales, etc.) and the age-set to which I am attached (preparing meals, joining in their entry to the annual fancy-dress competition, etc.). As some locals explicitly told me, by learning-through-doing I had shown a degree of openness which they respected and so, as far as I can judge, won for myself a certain level of acceptance. This continuing experience has also provided me with a diversity of overlapping contexts within which to attempt to understand what I have come to know about village ways and attitudes. As Malinowski pointed out decades ago, long-term fieldwork allows anthropologists to recognise some of the gaps between local rhetorics and realities; in my case, it has enabled me to ask locals how they try to reconcile the rift between the two. Also, because the main focus of my work was not directly on food, much of what I learnt was by observation and serendipity: unexpected events happening in front of me during the long course of my fieldwork, which I would then ask the locals to explain.

It is important to underline that I was not so much gradually gaining an idea of their way of life as collectively constructing with them a certain interpretation of the village. Clifford (1980) has spoken of the fieldwork encounter between anthropologist and key pundits as less a work of translation and more a joint production of an intercultural text. In other words, an anthropologist and his or her informants produce a series of questions and answers in which the interloper attempts to comprehend what his or her hosts are doing and why, while the locals are trying to understand the aims of their visitor and respond accordingly. In the process, both the questions and answers of the participants in this ongoing discussion become ever more refined, and the intersubjectivity they are creating that much more extensive and subtle. The result, according to Clifford, is not a definitive ethnography but a book which should be assessed as the complicit manufacture by the parties involved of a historically contingent intercultural text. On this reading, anthropologists do not simply discover 'what is going on in the village' but painstakingly help put together a collection of 'partial truths'.

Clifford's approach is itself all too obviously partial. It forgets the other conversations an ethnographer participates in before production of his or her ethnography: dialogues with colleagues and other academics, all of which help in the formulation of the partial truths. But Clifford's key point should still be well taken. Anthropologists do not deal in hard-edge facts which, like tins on a supermarket shelf, can be pulled down by a customer and rearranged as suits. The statements ethnographers fabricate are much more grounded, a fact they have to stress to some of their readers, who might otherwise be easily mislead.

## A Final Point

Anthropologists cannot prescribe exactly which food-related dimensions promoters of local identity may wish to focus on. They may stress particular foods, combinations of foods, particular prohibitions, styles of cooking, particular tastes or textures, structures and timing of meals, size of portions, table manners, and so on. It is up to the fieldworker to find out exactly which are being used to drive the vehicle of identity.

## References

Barth, F. (1969) Introduction. In Barth, F. (ed.) *Ethnic Groups and Boundaries: The social organization of culture difference*, Universitetsforlaget, Oslo: 9–38.
Boissevain, J. (ed.) (1992) *Revitalizing European Rituals*, Routledge, London.
Clifford, J. (1980) Fieldwork, Reciprocity, and the Making of Ethnographic Texts, *Man* 15: 518–532.
Eriksen, T.H. (1993) *Ethnicity and Nationalism: Anthropological perspectives*, Pluto, London.
Fragner, B. (2000) Social Reality and Culinary Fiction: the perspective of cookbooks from Iran and Central Asia. In Zubaida, S. and Tapper, R (eds.) *A Taste of Thyme: Culinary cultures of the Middle East*, Taurus, London: 63–71.
Hobsbawm, E., and Ranger, T. (eds.) (1983) *The Invention of Tradition*, Cambridge University Press, Cambridge.
MacClancy, J.V. (1996) Sport, Identity and Ethnicity. In MacClancy, J.V. (ed.) *Sport, Identity and Ethnicity*, Berg, Oxford: 1–20.

MacClancy, J.V. (1997) Anthropology, Art and Contest. In MacClancy, J.V. (ed.) *Contesting Art. Art, Politics and Identity in the Modern World,* Berg, Oxford: 1–26.

MacClancy, J.V. (n.d.) *Cultures of Nationalism: a Basque example.* Forthcoming.

Zubaida, S. (2000) National, Communal and Global Dimensions in Middle Eastern Food Cultures. In Zubaida, S. and Tapper, R. (eds.) *A Taste of Thyme: Culinary cultures of the Middle East,* Taurus, London: 33–45.

# 6. DOING IT WRONG
## WHY BOTHER TO DO IMPERFECT RESEARCH?

*Gerald Mars* and *Valerie Mars*

## The Problem

There is a big problem in advising anyone how to do research. And no less a problem in receiving advice. This is because so much advice is necessarily concerned with ideal methods and ideal standards. As a result, recipients are likely to become apprehensive before they get to the field, demoralised when in it and often despairing when they emerge to write up. This veneration of the ideal, is evident in a whole range of disciplines but perhaps especially so in social anthropology. This paper is concerned with its implications for studies in the social anthropology of food. We need to counter – or at least modify – this dangerous drive to the ideal!

The trouble with food is that it is so ephemeral. Here it is one minute – and gone the next. It is therefore easy to ignore food. But being ephemeral is also its strength. Though the eating of food may be ephemeral, its production, preparation and presentation is repetitive. It therefore has an independence – and its repetition can be studied independently. Understanding patterns of repetition can tell us much about a people's social organisation. If a structure can be thought of as made up of building blocks – then food and its context is the cement that shows how these blocks are bonded together. That is fine as far as it goes. But in planning and starting one's fieldwork, and particularly in the day to day doing of it, there are problems not often effectively addressed. What about changing track if the pre-planning does not work out? What if it is not possible to get adequate data? What if the data does not seem to make any theoretical or indeed any sort of sense? How in these circumstances do you get to grips with sorting out what might be the lesser from the more important data? These kinds of problem seem to be the essence of fieldwork.

## Three 'Rules'

Three rules that can usefully influence research methods will be developed here. Examples of how these have operated will then be offered from the authors' experiences in studying different aspects of the social anthropology of food

- The first rule is to 'follow your material wherever it may lead' (Marx 1967, pxii). Emmanuel Marx quotes this maxim of Max Gluckman. It means that when collecting material you need the freedom not to be dominated by pre-existing sociological models – nor indeed be concerned with constructing them. Both are 'short cuts to reality'. They necessarily involve disregarding data and suppressing material that might well prove vital in formulating later and different interpretations. But what to do if emerging data are overwhelming but appear to have nothing to do with your planned project, or divert you from following your research plan?
- The second rule is concerned with the idea of what is 'good enough': it involves accepting that the ideal is rarely attainable – and this applies to fieldwork more than to most other aspects of research. Instead we must accept a standard that, *in the circumstances,* is 'good enough'. It derives from Donald W. Winnicott, one of the fathers of modern psychoanalysis, who first raised the idea of 'good enough' standards (Winnicott and Winnicott 1982). However, it is very relevant to fieldwork in social anthropology. So, when we are told that we should ideally spend a full calendar year in the field we must accept that this is often impossible. When we are told that we have to speak the language of informants this too is an ideal that might not always be attainable. What do we do when it is not possible to cross-check our informants' accounts or we are not allowed to participate in their activities – or perhaps not even allowed to observe them?
- The third rule follows from the second. It involves not falling into the trap of imposing our own outside assessments on the actors we are studying but assessing them according to their own assessments. This is the classic etic/emic distinction, a variation on well-established warnings against ethnocentricity. Winnicott, for instance, was concerned that social workers and psychiatric professionals applied unrealistically high standards in their assessments of mothers they defined as 'inadequate'. But this was an outside, an etic assessment. What, in fact, was going on? Were a mother's standards considered adequate by her peers? Were the results adequate in the circumstances in which mothers found themselves? How would this mother be assessed by other mothers? Good questions but are emic assessments always so pure and etic ones always to be scrapped?

Two cases from the authors' fieldwork experiences will now be offered to illustrate the three rules and show how they influenced methods of data collection on the anthropology of food. The first involved the study of a family-run restaurant in northern Italy.

## Food, Food History and Gift-giving in Emilia Romagna, Italy

This was a project that negated most of the ideal research prescriptions and yet managed to come up with what we, at least, consider to be useful data. It illustrates all three 'rules'.

Emilia Romagna is noted for the excellence of its food. Parma ham, salami, parmesan cheese and balsamic vinegar are exported throughout the world. So when the chance came to study a Michelin starred family restaurant in Emilia Romana, famous for its traditional menu and with its own organic garden, and when the family offered access and eagerness to help, it was an opportunity to be grasped. Gerald Mars (GM) had studied several restaurants and was interested in how they might be organised. Valerie Mars (VM) was interested in the nature of food preparation and the history of cuisine. To study such a highly successful enterprise with the added dimension of seeing the dynamics of family organisation was extremely attractive. There were, however, drawbacks. Some were evident immediately, others emerged later.

The first obvious handicap was that neither of us had adequate Italian so it was necessary to have an interpreter, a friend of the restaurant-owning family. Further, this was a busy restaurant so it was inconvenient to enter the kitchen as an observer. Nor was it possible to participate in food preparation. Third, we could only go to Italy for short visits, only four and a half weeks in all. Finally, when we arrived for the first stint, the family decided that for their help and access, they wanted a *quid pro quo* – a history of their family, written as part of the deal. This would obviously involve long discursive interviews with each family member. And with limited time available this was a distinct problem. It meant intensive work with an interpreter who was beginning to act as a censor and proving reluctant to interpret fully material she felt might be damaging to the family. We therefore received what we could see was an extremely lopsided view of the family as an ideally harmonious unit and were not in position to check this against reality. Later internal evidence was indeed to discredit this ideal.

These were serious handicaps. We debated whether to abort the project but decided, with some reluctance, to carry on. First we would write the family history, though without enthusiasm. It was not an area we thought would be of much interest. What emerged, however, was an ethnographic gold mine – we learned not only about the traditional cuisine and role of food in earlier Emilia Romagna society but how it adapted to later social changes. The restaurant's menus were a lexicon: they charted the shift – from specific festival foods of the past and food given as gifts – to their presentation as staple restaurant fare. It was a route from ritual validation to the iconic food symbols that now define this region (Szathmary 1983), and which also served to validate the family's image of itself as ideally harmonious – an image that was central to their functioning.

Learning the family history was important in understanding traditional gender roles and ideas of social mobility that were still strong in underpinning this family's present ventures. Indeed much of what they did in the present was justified by perceptions and reiterations of the past. Prior to 1946 in this area of Emilia Romagna, agriculture had depended on landless labourers and small family farmers. Three or four generation extended families, based on the agnatic links of brothers, worked small mixed farms of about twelve hectares. Land tenure was based on sharecropping (Sereni 1997, Zamagni 1997). There were three principal grades of sharecropper who received a third or a half of the value of their produce depending on their ownership of livestock or their lack of it. Mobility was possible but difficult. It was effected in large part by obtaining credit to finance the first step from landless labourer on to and then up the sharecropping ladder. The final aspirational level was for a group of brothers to achieve full ownership of a farm with, of course, retention of all its produce. It was not possible to make more than one shift each generation. Land ownership, therefore, was not so much valued as revered.

The possibility of mobility by obtaining credit was based entirely on family reputation, a matter still of central concern. One important criterion was the family's collective and demonstrated ability to produce high quality foods. The quality of its products demonstrated a family's collective skills not only in growing and rearing its own raw materials but also in its control of processes and the skills it brought to them. In this way a family was able to demonstrate how it could work in unison as a skilled, harmonious and integrated group – qualities that carried considerable moral value. And they still do: the restaurant owning family was similarly very concerned to demonstrate their harmony in the present. These qualities were then assessed through appraisal of the regular flow of its produce given as gifts to the landlord (or his agent) and to the priest. They were vital to the mobility process. If we had not agreed to examine the family's history we could not have appreciated the nature of its collectivism or the importance still placed on giving gifts of food.

Discussing the family's history involved learning about roles and gender divisions on the farm, the way decisions were collectively arrived at, and the ways individualism was subverted to the family collectivity. We learned that short-term processes like the daily making of pasta was the preserve of women, whilst longer, and therefore, more expensive capital intensive production of ham, parmesan or salami, was the province of men. The same divisions of labour were still evident in the restaurant. So too were the same methods of collective decision making and the doubling up of skills so that every restaurant role had a reserve role holder – similar to the way skills had been ordered on the farm.

Particularly important in this past agricultural world was the place of festivals in the life both of the family and of the wider community. We were able to discuss the ritual and symbolic significance of festival foods and how these, with adaptation, were now manifest as standard menu items.

We came to appreciate why food in Emilia Romagna was, and still is, so important in that the drive to excellence could, on occasion, still defy the 'common sense' of market realities. But to get to this appreciation involved a long detour through the family's ideal past. The current production by the youngest son of its twenty-year-old Balsamic Vinegar for instance, is so labour and time intensive that its eventual capital appreciation makes no sense in terms of orthodox economics. As in the past, it is given by the family as a gift – but now to friends and the restaurant's special customers. Similarly, the special skills to produce a finely crafted ham, *Culatello*, are both rare and time consuming. The excellence of food is still, in part, rated on non-economic criteria in Emilia Romagna – it is rated in the personal and publicly accredited pride and reputation that follows the competitive production of the highest quality food. Just as in the days of sharecropping agriculture. And their phenomenally labour-intensive organic garden emerged as more than just a means to produce good food: it was the last link to their ancestral land.

If we had been satisfied with nothing less than the ideals of full participant observation; if we had felt our limited availability was inadequate and if lacking command of the native language had deterred us, then we would not have begun the project. If we had not gone where the research took us – into reconstructing the past and the role of food in the past – we should not have been able to appreciate the role of food in the present or really understood how the restaurant worked. We did the best we could in the circumstances available. Though these were admittedly far from ideal, we contend they were 'good enough'. Good enough here means that our findings are sufficiently coherent and consistent to be supplemented or countered by library research or developed by other field researchers with more time and perhaps better skills. Research is ongoing and always incomplete.

But shortly after our last field trip a tragedy, following a crisis in relationships within the family, resulted in the restaurant's closure and the family's dispersal. There are two implications. The first emphasises the need to reconsider the orthodox virtues associated with the emic viewpoint. Here it was concerned to project an ideal that was far removed from reality. The second was that if we had waited for a more propitious time a unique research opportunity would have been lost! The final lesson is that researchers always have to strike while the iron is hot!

## Feasts and the Black Economy in Soviet Georgia

This was a study that moved sideways into food in that food had no part in the initial field plan. It was initially devised as a study of the black or hidden economy of Soviet Georgia. Georgia, with an estimated 30 percent plus of illegal production, had by far the biggest percentage of black gross national product (GNP) in the Soviet Union (Grossman 1977, Wiles 1981). The problem was that the Soviet Union was disinclined, to put it mildly, to allow investigation of something it abhorred and denied existed.

Israel, however, has a sizeable community of expatriate Georgian Jews who had left within the previous seven years. It was decided, therefore, to study this community to try to find out how the Georgian second economy was organised. This was by no means an ideal method but it was hoped it might prove 'good enough'. Initially we had no interest in their feasts but as work proceeded it became evident that feasts were not only the cement that bonded Georgian social life: it was their feasts that enabled Georgians to bypass and oppose the Soviet Command economy (Mars and Altman 1987a). Feasts emerged as symbiotic with the working of both the formal and the black economies.

This study, however, very nearly never started. There were objections from anthropological assessors that these expatriates, being Jews, were unrepresentative of their non-Jewish compatriots. It was also asserted that they were not 'real' Georgians at all and anyway their experiences were too much in the past to be reliable. There was also an objection that the study was based on retrospection and not on contemporary participant observation.

Then, GM was able to visit Soviet Georgia as an exchange scholar for a few brief weeks. Being regarded as a spy, however, seriously limited access to data, but he did attend several feasts. GM and VM also attended Israeli-Georgian feasts. They were not of especial interest to us in the early stages of fieldwork. VM, as a female foreigner, was categorised as an honorary man and this unfortunately precluded her having contact with the women preparing and serving the food.

There were three phases to the fieldwork in Israel. The first was to carry out a straightforward anthropological field study and, when this was established, to attempt to determine how far Jewish social organisation in Israel differed from that of non-Jewish Georgians back in Georgia. The aim was to see whether there had been significant differences between them. Yochannan Altman, an Israeli, was appointed as a research assistant and he did most of the Israeli fieldwork speaking Ivrit (modern Hebrew) rather than Georgian. We found that in Georgia differences between Jewish and non-Jewish Georgians had been much less than might have been expected. One difference was that admittedly Jews had been endogamous, another was that they drank less than non-Jewish Georgians. In Israel, though, they were beginning to drink more than they had done and considerably more than other Israelis. But there had been little anti-Semitism in Georgia, perhaps because Georgians tended to focus their discrimination on resident Armenians. Accordingly, Jews were allowed to work in a wide range of jobs and Jewish males were often bonded as blood brothers to Georgians in what were often significant relationships for exploiting the black economy. The assessors' objections had been based on ideal prescriptions.

The second phase was to translate our understanding of observed social processes in Israel in an attempt to gain retrospective understanding of social and economic life back in Georgia. The third phase was then to deepen the analysis to gain retrospective understanding of Georgia's black economy organisation. This was done by building up closely cross-checked case studies, accounts of black economy production and distribution (Mars and Altman 1987b) involving different individuals at different positions in the same organisations. In each of these phases, however, feasts seemed to intrude not only into accounts of social life back in Georgia but into the day to day experience of collecting data in Israel.

Georgians are extremely hospitable. Feasting often got in the way of regular data collection. Georgian feasts are famous for excess, for the amount of alcohol consumed and the numbers involved. Feasts might be for only ten or twenty people, but feasts of a thousand were not uncommon in Soviet Georgia. The authorities tried to stop them on the grounds that they misused scarce resources and these were often stolen from the State (Ma'ariv 1982). It was only by attending feasts that understanding of their wider significance became evident, and then we realised the reasons for official disapproval.

Georgia is an honour and shame culture. Descent is through males with an emphasis on the solidarity and mutual obligations of brothers. Within family groups spheres of action are well defined, do not overlap and are non-competitive. Beyond the family, however, these limitations are reversed: insecurity, instability and perpetual re-ranking is the norm (Peristany 1966). Men thus have continuously to extend and maintain their networks, demonstrate manliness, 'to be *catso*', seek visible achievement, consume and, most importantly, display. Women too need to develop their networks. Giving and attending feasts facilitated these aims.

Georgians, in both Israel and Georgia, whether Jewish or not, will organise a feast on any of a wide range of pretexts: some are planned months in advance, others are spontaneous. The visit of a foreigner, a meeting with someone previously out of touch, a family *rite de passage,* the celebration or prospect of a business deal, all would be celebrated with a feast. Participation is normally restricted to men though this was less so in the more intellectual and cosmopolitan circles of Tblisi. Whatever their justifying pretext or size, feasts are examples of conspicuous consumption and display (Mars and Altman 1987c).

Women in both locations prepare the food and to do it the wife of the host mobilises help and resources from her network of women friends and relatives. In this way she too demonstrates the potency and extent of her network – particularly in her ability to prepare a spontaneous feast. Women will bring the food from the kitchen on very small plates – only five or six inches across – and at first these will be placed down the centre of the table. Before they can be emptied, however, more full plates are brought so that soon the table will be covered. Newly arriving plates are then stacked on earlier ones so that a table may be four or five plates deep by the evening's end. At the end of the feast the women clear away and redistribute the leftover food among themselves for their families and, on their return home, to the women in their networks who helped them in their preparations. The ramifications, the web of obligations and reciprocities of a single feast, can therefore be extensive. All of this would have been missed if we had not followed the data.

Despite their varying size the structure of feasts is always the same. Each feast has a 'Head of Table', the *Tamada,* who is not necessarily the host but who must be a person of authority. He orders the proceedings, offers toasts that punctuate and structure the feast – there are normally about twenty toasts – and he finally closes the feast when a toast is offered honouring him. Toasts serve to link and integrate. The first toasts honour those who are the putative cause of the gathering, a new graduate, a visitor, a business partner. Then toasts are made to idealise values and levels of social organisation above the level of the personal network. Both are brought together and made concrete through the personalities present. Thus toasts are offered 'To The Land of Georgia', and if foreigners are attending, to the lands of their countries also. If staffs of different institutions are present these institutions too will be toasted. There is thus a focusing through individuals of ideal and abstract valuations on the one hand and, by treating individuals as representatives, a linking of organis-ations on the other.

Near the end of the evening toasts might well become so abstract that they cover everyone and everything, such as toasts 'to the divine spirit', or 'to all in our land'. Or they become so specific that to a sober celebrant (and it is un-likely that there will be many of these), they appear quite silly, like drinking 'to the electric light without which we wouldn't be able to see what we are doing here'. This is when competitive drinking might well take over. Compe-tition is accentuated since men are not expected to relieve themselves and must stay in the room to obviate private urinating, purging or vomiting. Again, this is not a feature of cosmopolitan Tbilisi.

At the end of the feast, friendships are sworn, men may well eat from the same plate and drink from the same cup (known as *megobarebi* 'close friends') and it is then that addresses or cards are exchanged and networks formally con-solidated for possible future use. At one feast in Georgia GM exchanged cards with a fellow diner and said how honoured he had been to attend. The reply was insightful, if deflating: 'Huh – it's not the first feast that's important. It's the second!' – another insight into networking that would not have been gained without attending the feast.

When planning this study there had been no intention to take particular notice of feasts: but they intruded, so they *had* to be noticed. Gradually it became evident that the feast, as an institution with a long history, was more than a meal writ large and more than mere celebration. As a flexible and responsive cultural resource, the feast was part of a long and adaptive tra-dition. In Soviet Georgia it linked and bound people of different affiliations who represented different places, institutions, occupations and kinship link-ages. It was by developing and manipulating these ego-focused networks that Georgians were able to influence and manipulate the Soviet State to such a degree that Georgia became a byword for economic subversion.

The network – made manifest in the feast – served many functions. Networks, and the feasts, which maintained and expanded them, were necessary to smooth the path of Georgia's citizens at the numerous points of contact that linked them to myriad state organisations. They were not only vital in getting scarce goods but also in obtaining preferred jobs, acquiring permits and licenses, securing places at university and in smoothing out difficulties with the police and other authorities; feasting emerged as symbiotic with both the formal and informal economies.

One of the strengths of anthropology is that it encourages holism. This should in turn encourage a drive to 'follow the material' and if not seek connections, then at least embrace them when, serendipitously, they present themselves. An economist's analysis of Georgia's black economy would have been unlikely to uncover the significance of the feast just as an economist would not have appreciated the 'uneconomic' production of foods in Emilia Romagna. But the claims of anthropological orthodoxy were adamant: one must be directly involved in participant observation with the people one is concerned to know. If the authorities preclude fieldwork, then you have no project. But invariably, if ideals cannot be met there are alternatives, not perfect ones perhaps, but ones that might well prove 'good enough'. We like to think that, as one result, a new approach to 'retrospective fieldwork' was able to be added to the tools available to social anthropology.

## Overall

We have presented two attenuated case studies to demonstrate the working of what might pretentiously be called 'rules' and to show the methods we adopted to study different aspects of the anthropology of food. In Emilia Romagna, food featured from the beginning. But the methods used had to be circuitous: the present was only revealed by recourse to the past. In the study of Soviet Georgia's black economy, food initially had no place – but it intruded and its centrality became significant as the study progressed: the past was explicable only through study of the present. Here too, the repetitious nature of food and its associated relationships emerged as central to understanding the principles that underlie social organisation.

Both approaches diverged from orthodox field methods: each involved following the material and going where it led; adapting methods and aims to their context and abandoning injunctions to follow ideals by embracing the 'good enough'. Researchers may not immediately appreciate the value of some of the data they find. It would be surprising if they did. The data may not seem to make a lot of sense – they rarely do – but they might do later. The data may appear, or even be, fragmentary and incomplete. This is often the case, especially early on in fieldwork. Nonetheless, researchers should record information as it arises. Some pieces of data may not be immediately useful, but may well click into place later, sometimes much later. And this keeps the door open to new understandings in a way that questionnaire studies or other forms of rigid sociological frameworks never can.

The too slavish following of 'a ready-made sociological mould' also has implications when analysing data and writing up on return from the field. It applies, of course, not only to food. GM well recalls Professor Raymond Firth, his PhD supervisor at the time, showing exasperation as he explained his difficulties in writing up his research – it did not fit the theoretical frame GM thought it should. 'Look' said Firth, 'never mind the theoretical frame. Write in the first instance as if you're writing an account for your auntie. Then let the theory emerge from the data' – advice we have found invaluable ever since and as these cases have, we hope, revealed.

This maxim to 'follow the material', offers further insights. It means being prepared to follow new directions when these present themselves. It means embracing serendipity – even, and especially, if you do not know where it will lead. It means following lines of enquiry that might not have seemed relevant at the initial fieldwork planning stage. Many invaluable and exciting insights have been garnered by following serendipitous opportunities that presented themselves when least expected.

Fieldworkers have to make do with those methods that the context allows. We would all like to spend longer in the field, especially if limited to less than the traditionally prescribed full calendrical year. We know that ideally we should speak the native language of our informants and not rely on interpreters – especially if we distrust the accounts they might be giving us. We know we should cross-check information with different informants and should participate in a variety of different ways if we are to understand them fully. But what should we do if one or more of these conditions cannot be met? Do we abort the research exercise because the preconditions are not perfect? In real life preconditions are very rarely perfect – though you might not think so from reading the polished accounts that emerge in reports, papers and books.

Every shift from the ideal offers the chance of new material and new insights. If we target our research to food we might be able to stay on target – or we may not. It might be that the route to knowledge about food proves more circuitous than we had thought. We recall a postgraduate student who returned in dejection from South America. She had been unable to enter the territory of her chosen people because of the avaricious demands of officials who controlled access. Their demands for bribes had exhausted her budget. Not for her was there a chance to study food – or anything else. Her supervisor was furious. What a wonderful opportunity she had missed – to make a study of bribery! And who knows what she might have uncovered about the food ways of bribe takers?

## Acknowledgements

We are grateful to Dr Leonard Mars for commentary on this chapter as well as to Gillian Riley for our introduction to the family and restaurant in Emilia Romagna, and for interpreting and translation.

## References

Grossman, G. (1977) The Second Economy of USSR, *Problems of Communism*, Sept/Oct: 25–40.

Ma'ariv (Israeli evening paper) (1982), Georgian hospitality under attack, *Ma'ariv*, September 6th, Tel Aviv.

Mars, G. and Altman, Y. (1987a) Alternative mechanism of distribution in a Soviet economy. In Douglas, M. (ed.) *Constructive Drinking: perspectives on drink from anthropology*, Cambridge University Press, Cambridge: 270–279.

Mars, G. and Altman, Y. (1987b) Case studies in second economy production and transportation in Soviet Georgia. In Alessandrini, S. and Dallago, B. (eds) *The Unofficial Economy*, Gower Publishing, Aldershot: 197–218.

Mars, G. and Altman, Y. (1987c) Case studies in second economy distribution in soviet Georgia. In Alessandrini, S. and Dallago, B. (eds) *The Unofficial Economy*, Gower Publishing, Aldershot: 219–246.

Marx, E. (1967) *Bedouin of the Negev*, Manchester University Press, Manchester.

Peristiany, J.G. (1966) Introduction. In Peristiany, J.G. (ed.) *Honour and Shame*, Weidenfeld and Nicholson, London: 9–18.

Sereni, E. (1997) *History of the Italian Agricultural Landscape*, (translated by R. Burr Litchfield), Princeton University Press, Princeton, New Jersey.

Szathmary, L. (1983) How festive foods of the Old World became commonplace in the New, or the American perception of Hungarian goulash: food in motion. In *The Migration of Foodstuffs and Cookery Techniques*, Proceedings of The Oxford Symposium, Volume 1., Prospect Books, London: 137–143.

Wiles, P. (1981) *Die Parallelwietschaft*, Sonderveroffentlichung des Bundesinstituts für Ostwissenschaftliche und Internationale Studien, Cologne.

Winnicott, D.W. and Winnicott, C. (1982) *Playing and Reality,* Routledge, London.

Zamagni, V. (1997) *The Economic History of Italy, 1860–1990*, Clarendon Press, Oxford.

# 7. METHODS FOR ASSESSING TASTE ABILITIES AND HEDONIC RESPONSES IN HUMAN AND NONHUMAN PRIMATES

*Bruno Simmen, Patrick Pasquet* and *Claude Marcel Hladik*

## Introduction

As a primary interface between an organism and the alimentary environment, the taste system is a major part of the physiological background from which feeding behaviour and food habits have developed. Accordingly, investigating taste abilities helps us understand not only the former interface that shaped the present human condition, but how sociocultural parameters currently interact with such a background as well. From an evolutionary perspective, nonhuman primates provide a reliable model for the study of the relationships between food choices and taste abilities. According to this logic, investigation of the large variability of human feeding behaviour should start from a similar biological basis and the possibility of its variation in different human populations, before one embarks on assessing cross-cultural variation.

## Taste Parameters

Most studies on taste abilities have focused on three main parameters: taste quality, taste intensity and pleasantness/unpleasantness of taste. In taste tests, the use of pure compounds in solutions allows one to focus on the gustatory component of the taste sensation. But one should note that the taste sensation elicited by food generally involves a multimodal sensory response including taste, olfaction and tactile stimulation. This complex perception results from the convergence between taste and olfactory processing into the brain cortex (Rolls 1997). It is not our intention here to provide an exhaustive review of methods used to characterise human taste perception, given the plethora of methods (e.g. Bartoshuk 1978, Meilgaard *et al.* 1987). Instead only basic methods, relevant to the topic of sensory anthropology, will be presented.

Gustatory perception is usually assessed by a measurement of taste thresholds (i.e. the minimum perceived concentration of a taste stimulus) and suprathreshold taste responses (i.e. the perceived intensity and hedonic dimension). These involve distinct methodological approaches in nonhuman primates and in humans.

## Methods for Studying Taste in Nonhuman Primates

In primates, the recording of taste responses is based on a spontaneous choice of the solutions provided. Accordingly, the taste response is necessarily global, including recognition together with acceptance/rejection of the stimulus, at the threshold level and above the threshold.

The procedure designed for determining taste threshold in primates, the two-bottle test, was initially used by Glaser (1968), following the pioneering work of Richter and Campbell (1939) on rodents. A solution of a compound (for instance sucrose) is presented simultaneously with a bottle of water and the spontaneous consumption of each liquid is recorded. Various concentrations of the compound are presented, up to the lowest concentration at which there is no difference in the consumption of water and tested solution.

This procedure has been modified by Simmen and Hladik (1988), using a random presentation of the various concentrations and applying a statistical test (paired-sample t-test) to determine the lowest concentration for which a significant difference of consumption occurs. The time of each test is limited to a short period (ranging from a few minutes to three hours, according to the substance and the average body weight of the species tested), because any long-term post-ingestive effect might affect ingestive response. This is especially true when testing sugar solutions. Furthermore, the test should be performed before the animals are fed with their daily meal.

The position of the two bottles must be varied at random during each trial, to avoid a side-preference effect, especially during a period of familiarisation at the beginning of the test. Tests are started after completing a period of habituation during which the individuals are supplied with a high concentration of sugar solution and tap water simultaneously. Habituation is considered achieved when a marked preference for the sweet solution is recorded over four successive trials.

This type of test can be used for both attractive substances (sugars) and distasteful compounds (such as quinine or tannins); however, using the latter type to determine taste rejection thresholds necessitates a maintenance of the animal's motivation by providing, alternately, a sweet solution at suprathreshold concentration. An alternative protocol for distasteful compounds is to mix the tastant with a moderately sweet solution (twice the threshold), to be provided simultaneously with the same sweet solution, instead of water (Simmen *et al.* 1999). This procedure is particularly appropriate for tannin solutions, which are subject to oxidation, as it reduces the duration of the tests.

Such thresholds, although determined by a behavioural method (that could imply weak responsiveness to low concentrations), have been compared with the sensitivity as measured on the peripheral nerve of the taste system. For instance, a tannic acid concentration of 0.13 g/l, applied on the tongue of mouse lemurs (*Microcebus murinus*) elicits a weak signal on the *chorda tympani* proper nerve, while the lowest behavioural response is observed for 0.19 g/l (Hellekant *et al.* 1993, Iaconelli and Simmen 1999). Accordingly, the two-bottle test is a reliable method for estimating taste thresholds.

The supra-threshold responses are recorded with similar protocols: the profile of supra-threshold responses is determined by plotting the amount of solution ingested against levels of concentration. The resulting profiles may resemble an asymmetric bell-shaped curve in the case of responses to sugar. In this case linear regression models can be applied to the increasing and the decreasing parts of the profile (after transforming data into their decimal logarithms); alternatively, the profiles may tend towards an asymptote for the inhibitory responses to tannins.

To categorise the taste qualities perceived by a primate, another type of behavioural method is required, based on conditioning. For instance, conditioned taste aversion towards sugars is obtained by injecting lithium chloride into the abdominal cavity, immediately after the animal consumed a sweet solution. The nausea provoked by lithium chloride is associated with the taste after one trial, and the animal will avoid any sweet-tasting compound in subsequent choice tests. In this case the notion of 'sweet' refers to human perception and the corresponding semantic descriptor. In the case of a primate, such as *Microcebus*, the animal will react negatively to any substance the taste of which resembles that of the conditioned stimulus. This method has been used to determine, within a panel of substances tasting sweet to humans, which ones were also perceived as 'sweet' by a primate (Hellekant et al. 1993).

## Taste Thresholds in Human Populations

In the research field of nutritional anthropology, a proper selection of the method for assessing taste abilities is paramount. The method for determining perception thresholds has been widely used in early studies of taste in humans. This method has many variants but generally involves two phases of testing.

An approximate detection threshold is first measured by providing various concentrations of a given compound, following an ascending or descending order (e.g. Harris and Kalmus 1949, Dixon and Massey 1969), and asking subjects whether they perceive a taste sensation different from that of water. A complementary test is then designed to check whether subjects are able to discriminate between water and solutions containing the concentration corresponding to this detection threshold. In this last phase, subjects are informed of the taste quality that they are supposed to discriminate from water. This method, which only involves discrimination against pure water, without recognition, has often been used to determine detection threshold in single-compound studies.

An alternative procedure, however, is more relevant to the topics of nutritional anthropology which address the issue of taste as a determinant of food intake. Food selection necessarily involves recognition of taste stimuli elicited by foods in the oral cavity. In this respect, taste recognition thresholds have to be assessed. The method for this differs from that mentioned above because a set of compounds is generally tested rather than a single substance, and so, more importantly, subjects must recognise taste qualities of the various substances. Accordingly, this reduces the influence of random responses.

Under laboratory controlled situations, the use of de-ionised or poorly mineralised water to prepare the solutions has been recommended. However, under field conditions, it is often more realistic to use local drinking water as subjects are used to the peculiar taste of their own water sources. The powders for each product should be weighed precisely and, for research in the field, it is a good idea to take ready-measured and labelled packets. As an example, for a test with a series of solutions at twofold steps of increasing concentration, each series is created starting with the highest concentration; each sample is diluted in a beaker with 100 ml of water, using a magnetic agitator. A volume of 50 ml of this solution is then poured into the first numbered flask and the remainder is diluted again with 50 ml of water and so on until a series of flasks is created. The resulting dilutions for a selection of taste tests are shown below (Table 7.1).

The solutions may have smaller or larger, but constant, intervals of dilution than in this example. Each solution should be carried without delay to the place where the tests will be carried out and left there to reach the ambient temperature. Solutions should be renewed regularly and this especially applies

***Table 7.1*** A selection of appropriate taste test solutions (twofold steps)

| |
|---|
| *For fructose: 11 dilutions from 1 to 1,000 millimoles per litre.* |
| *For sucrose: 9 dilutions from 1.5 to 400 millimoles per litre.* |
| *For sodium chloride: 10 dilutions from 0.5 to 250 millimoles per litre.* |
| *For citric acid: 8 dilutions from 0.2 to 25 millimoles per litre.* |
| *For quinine hydrochloride: 11 dilutions from 0.4 to 400 micromoles per litre.* |
| *For tannic acid: 12 dilutions from 4 to 8,000 micromoles per litre.* |
| *For oak tannin: 10 dilutions from 0.023 to 12 grams per litre.* |
| *For 6-n-propylthiouracil (PROP): 12 solutions from 1.9 to 3,800 micromoles per litre.* |

to the tannins, which are very unstable. A film will appear on the surface after a few hours, similar to what you see on a cup of tea that has been left to stand.

This test procedure (Hladik *et al.* 1986) is derived from the staircase method described by Cornsweet (1962). After informing the subject of the taste categories he or she could be faced with, such as water, salty, sour, sweet, bitter or astringent, recognition thresholds are measured during a blind test, in which the order of presentation of compounds is not known by the subjects. Solutions of tastants, prepared as explained above, are presented in a semi-randomised order (Figure 7.1), starting with the weakest solution in the order of increasing equal steps of concentrations. Substances like astringent tannins, the perception of which is likely to persist for a long period and might affect the sensitivity toward other substances, are generally given as the last stimuli within the set of compounds tested. Once the taste of two successive concentrations is recognised successfully, the subject is given the previous unrecognised solution (first reversal). This up-and-down procedure is performed twice until the taste of two increasing stimuli is correctly named. The actual recognition threshold is calculated as the arithmetic mean of the lowest concentrations recognised in each reversal.

This procedure gives a conservative estimate of the recognition thresholds. Other up-and-down procedures provide probabilistic figures, in which incorrect responses and correct responses allow the calculation of thresholds (Dixon and Massey 1969).

***Figure 7.1*** Blind tests for determining taste recognition thresholds (Photograph by F. Aubaile)

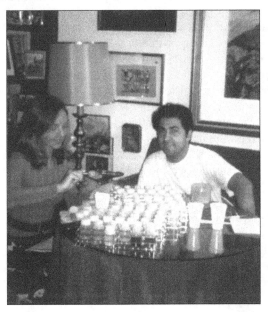

A one-minute interval after water rinses is necessary before presenting further solutions. Rinsing the tongue with the same water as is used for the dilutions allows subjects to remain in contact with a reference solution before assessing the taste of proposed stimuli. At the group/population level, the median threshold can be calculated using probit analysis (Finney 1971) after clustering individual thresholds into discrete classes of concentrations. The use of median thresholds rather than mean thresholds is appropriate for some compounds like the bitter tasting 6-$n$-propylthiouracil (PROP), the perception of which follows a bimodal distribution (see below).

A third parameter that has been used in studies of sensory psychophysiology is the taste discrimination threshold. This measures the ability of subjects to discriminate the smallest variation of concentration from a reference solution (Weber ratio). Following the method of constant stimuli described in Galanter (1962), subjects are provided with pairs of stimuli, of which one is the reference concentration. Subjects are asked to say which of the two stimuli is the strongest. Pairs may be delivered in ascending order (Laing et al. 1993), or by selecting four increments below and four increments above the reference concentration, with equidistant steps (Johansson et al. 1973). Within each pair, solutions are presented in a randomised order. Several reference concentrations can be used, since discrimination thresholds vary with the level of concentration. By convention, the threshold, or the 'just noticeable difference', is determined as the concentration variation that is perceived by 50 percent of the individuals.

## Measuring Taste Perception at a Supra-threshold Level

Apart from threshold measurements, it is particularly useful to characterise taste perception in terms of supra-threshold responses to stimuli. At this supra-threshold level, one asks the subject to distinguish between the intensity of the taste quality perceived and the hedonic value associated with that taste. The perception of taste intensity, as for thresholds, is globally less dependent upon affective and cognitive factors than the hedonic value of gustatory stimuli.

There are many variants of the methods used to assess taste intensity, many of which are based on the use of scales. Typically, subjects indicate on labelled scales or magnitude scales the intensity perceived when tasting a compound in solution. As for other sensory measurements, the presentation of stimuli should follow a random order or an increasing or decreasing concentration order. At least two trials of the same series should be performed.

As for labelled scales, a 5-point scale was originally introduced by Likert (1932), but it is now more common to use 9- or even 11-point scales, displayed vertically or horizontally (Figure 7.2). Responses are converted to scores on a scale ranging, for instance, from 1 (extremely weak) to 9 (extremely strong). The mean of individual scores is taken to provide an overall population score.

***Figure 7.2***    Example of a vertical 9-point labelled scale

How strong is the taste of this solution?

☐  extremely strong

☐  very strong

☐  strong

☐  slightly strong

☐  neutral

☐  slightly weak

☐  weak

☐  very weak

☐  extremely weak

Another scale designed to rate taste intensities, utilising descriptive words, is a semantically labelled scale of sensation magnitude (LMS) (Green *et al.* 1993). Unlike previous scales, the scale is continuous and avoids ceiling effects (e.g. responses to concentrated stimuli tend to aggregate towards the top anchor of the scale). It also represents an absolute scale of perceived intensity while taking into account subject-specific intensity magnitude estimates. This scale is composed of six verbal semantic descriptors from *barely detectable* to *strongest imaginable* taste according to the geometric means of their rated magnitudes (Figure 7.3).

Taste hedonics is investigated using either labelled or visual analogue scales. When using analogue scales, the pleasantness or the unpleasantness of the sensation for a given stimulus is expressed by the subject, with a stroke on a line anchored with *maximal pleasure* at one end and *maximal displeasure* at the other end. In some cases, a sign indicating *indifference* is displayed in the middle of the line. Also, subjects are allowed to express extreme responses beyond the visual limits of the scale. This occurs, for instance, when a stimulus is judged more pleasant or more unpleasant compared with a concentration previously evaluated as eliciting maximal displeasure or pleasure (Figure 7.4). This hedonic or affective response is then translated into numeric values by measuring the distance (in mm) between the stroke and the *indifference* point. Positive values represent pleasant sensations and negative values unpleasant ones.

***Figure 7.3***   The oral labelled magnitude scale (after Green et al. 1993)

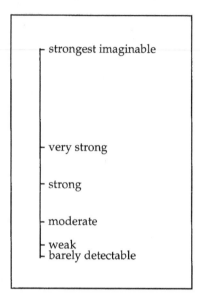

***Figure 7.4***   Visual analogue scale for hedonic rating

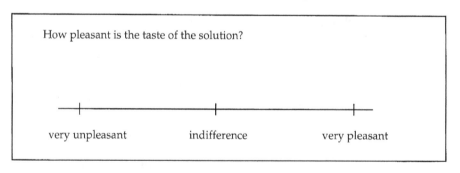

Visual analogue scales offer possibilities to assess taste hedonics in populations including non-literate informants or school children. An alternative is to use a faces scale in which a 7-point scale is replaced by stylised faces figuring expressions from joy to gloom (Andrews and Withey 1976). Subjects are then asked to say which face is the closest to what they feel when tasting a solution. Stylised faces may be limited to represent only the extremities of the scale, e.g. a 'grimacing face with tongue protruding' at the left hand and 'happy face licking its lips' at the other end, which correspond respectively to the terms 'not liked at all' and 'liked a lot' (Looy and Weingarten 1992).

Scales labelled with varying numbers of points are often used to assess hedonic responses (e.g. Peryam and Pilgrim 1957). However, using this type of scale may be hampered by the ceiling effects, which, as is the case for taste intensity, reduce the discrimination among the most liked or disliked foods. The Labelled Affective Magnitude (LAM) scale, proposed by Schutz and Cardello (2001) allows one to circumvent this effect and to distinguish subgroups (Pasquet *et al.*, 2002). This scale is an 11-point vertical scale with *greatest imaginable pleasure* and *greatest imaginable displeasure* at each end (Figure 7.5). The response (a bar on the scale) is measured positively, or negatively, from midway, to be re-scaled from –100 to +100 between the two extreme semantic labels (see also Macbeth and Mowatt, this volume).

Another technique has been developed to investigate neonate taste responses or as an alternative to the use of hedonic scales. This technique is based on the evidence that humans as well as nonhuman primates display a gusto-facial reflex when in contact with concentrated taste stimuli. Such behaviour occurs rapidly after the stimulus is presented. In this method, facial expressions in response to the application of a taste stimulus on the tongue are recorded using a video tape. The method has been used in early studies of taste among nonhuman primates, including infants, and among human neonates (Steiner 1977, Steiner and Glaser1984). It also allows one to circumvent possible cognitive or culturally determined attitudes which may arise when subjects are asked to judge solutions. More recently, it has been applied to categorise mimics expressed by young adults in response to sweet substances (Looy and Weingarten 1992). In this test, a panel of adults is asked to decide from videotapes figuring subject

*Figure 7.5* Labelled Affective Magnitude (LAM) scale (after Schutz and Cardello 2001)

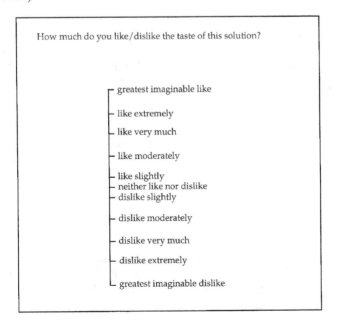

responses to taste stimuli, whether subjects like, are neutral to or dislike the solution proposed. They indicate on a 5-point scale how confident they feel about their judgement.

## A Screening Method Applied to the Investigation of Perception of PTC/PROP Substances

The genetically determined ability to taste the bitter substances, 6-$n$-propyl-thiouracil (PROP) and phenylthiocarbamide (PTC), has received considerable attention in the literature of genetics, anthropology and sensory physiology. Early studies used the bimodal distribution of sensitivity (tasters vs. non-tasters) in populations as a marker to study human genetic diversity (for a review see Hladik and Pasquet 1999).

More recently, investigations of PROP/PTC tasting have been aimed at understanding the relationship between genetically determined taste sensitivity and the development of taste preferences and food use (Drewnowski and Rock 1995). For such studies, Bartoshuk (1993) used a three-group typology according to PROP sensitivity (respectively non-tasters, tasters and a group of highly sensitive individuals, the super-tasters). These groups are distinguished according to PROP detection thresholds within a range of fifteen PROP solutions (1.0 – 3,200 micromoles per litre) incremented in quarter-log steps. After separating tasters and non-tasters (cut-point at 0.2 millimoles per litre), the super-tasters are then identified among the tasters on the basis of the mean ratio of intensity of supra-threshold intensity rating PROP solutions relative to sodium chloride solutions.

A rapid and simplified screening method has been developed by Drewnowski *et al.* (1997) to avoid such a long testing process in population-based studies. In this method the subjects are asked to place PROP-impregnated filter paper (dried after impregnation with a saturated PROP solution) on the back of the tongue, let it get moist and rate the bitterness on a 9-point category scale (from 1 = *not at all bitter* to 9 = *extremely bitter*). The subjects are then divided into three groups, respectively those who rated the paper 1 or 2, those who rated it 3–7, and those who rated it 8 or 9. A cross-validation (Monneuse *et al.* 2000) showed that the simplified method of Drewnowski *et al.* (1997) yielded results quite comparable to those obtained with the series of PROP solutions, thus permitting the discrimination between 'non-tasters', 'tasters' and 'super-tasters'.

## Conclusion

Methods for assessing taste perception in both nonhuman primates and humans are provided in this chapter because anthropologists interested in the evolution of sensory systems and related literature need to be aware of methodological differences and associated terms. In particular, thresholds can be measured with different techniques and these do not necessarily provide similar meanings for sensory studies in both humans and nonhuman primates.

The issues addressed are crucial for choosing between techniques. For instance in both nonhuman primates and humans, detection thresholds can be measured . For nonhuman primates a conditioned taste procedure can be used and for humans one can record verbal responses to tasting solutions (blind test). The resulting thresholds may be compared, especially if the aim of the study is to relate food selection to taste sensitivity.

In practice, one should be careful that subjects do not experience sensory fatigue, which imposes limitations on the number of tests that can be performed. For instance, when determining recognition thresholds, the use of five or six different compounds is a maximum recommended for investigations. Another fact which must be borne in mind is that trained subjects give better performances than naïve subjects when tasting solutions (Pangborn 1959). Accordingly, repeated measures may yield different values. This phenomenon, however, is reduced when tests are based on recognition of taste qualities instead of on measuring 'just-noticeable differences' or taste detection thresholds.

Technically, one should be aware that the gustatory parameters measured are sensitive to sampling bias and variability, especially parameters involving hedonic aspects. It is thus recommended that researchers carry out tests on relatively homogenous groups, differentiated, for example, by sex, age, smoker/ non smoker status, pathology, hormonal status, state of hunger or other satiety factors (e.g. Bourlière *et al.* 1958, Whissell-Buechy 1990, Bartoshuk *et al.* 1996, Bartoshuk 2000). One should recall, for example, the lowered perception of food taste during rhinitis (e.g. the common cold), although this particularly affects the smell component of the oral sensation instead of the taste perception. With regard to methods aimed at measuring taste intensities or hedonics, one should be cautious about scales, especially those which include verbal descriptors, as these may not necessarily be universally suited for cross-cultural comparisons or across age categories (see Macbeth and Mowatt this volume).

# References

Andrews, F.M. and Withey, S.B. (1976) *Social Indicators of Well-being: Americans' perception of life quality*, Plenum Press, New York.

Bartoshuk, L.M. (1978) The psychophysics of taste, *American Journal of Clinical Nutrition*, 31: 1068–1077.

Bartoshuk, L.M. (1993) The biological basis of food perception and acceptance, *Food Quality and Preference*, 4: 21–32.

Bartoshuk, L.M. (2000) Hormones, age, genes and pathology: how do we assess variation in sensation and preference? *European Journal of Clinical Nutrition*, 54: S4.

Bartoshuk, L.M., Duffy, V.B., Reed, D. and Williams, A. (1996) Supertasting, earaches and head injury: genetics and pathology alter our taste worlds, *Neuroscience and Biobehavioral Reviews*, 20: 79–87.

Bourlière, F., Cendron, H. and Rapaport, A. (1958) Modification avec l'âge des seuils gustatifs de perception et de reconnaissance aux saveurs salée et sucrée, chez l'homme, *Gerontologia*, 2: 104–112.

Cornsweet, T.N. (1962) The staircase-method in psychophysics, *American Journal of Psychology*, 75: 485–491.

Dixon, W. and Massey, F. (1969) *Introduction to statistical analyses*, 3rd edition, MacGraw Hill Company, New York

Drewnowski, A. and Rock, C.L. (1995) The influence of genetic taste markers on food acceptance, *American Journal of Clinical Nutrition*, 62: 506–511.

Drewnowski , A. Henderson, S.A. and Shore, A.B. (1997) Genetic sensitivity to 6-n-propylthiouracil (PROP) and hedonic responses to bitter and sweet tastes, *Chemical Senses*, 22: 27–37.

Finney, D.J. (1971) *Probit analyses. A statistical treatment of the sigmoid response curve*, 3rd edition, Cambridge University Press, Cambridge.

Galanter, E. (1962) Contemporary psychophysics. In Brown, R., Galanter, E., Hess, E.H. and Mandler, G. (eds) *New Directions in Psychology*, Holt, Rinehart and Winston, New York: 87–156.

Glaser, D. (1968) Geschmacksschwellenwerte bei Callithricidae (Platyrrhina), *Folia Primatologica*, 9: 246–257.

Green, B.G., Shaffer, G.S. and Gilmore, M.M. (1993) Derivation and evaluation of a semantic scale of oral sensation magnitude with apparent ratio properties, *Chemical Senses*, 18: 683–702.

Harris, H. and Kalmus, H. (1949) The measurement of taste sensitivity to phenylthiourea (PTC), *Annals of Eugenics*, 15: 24–31.

Hellekant, G., Hladik, C.M., Dennys, V., Simmen, B., Roberts, T.W., Glaser, D., DuBois, G. and Walters, D.E. (1993) On the sense of taste in two Malagasy primates (*Microcebus murinus* and *Eulemur mongoz*), *Chemical Senses*, 18: 307–320.

Hladik, C.M. and Pasquet, P. (1999) Evolution des comportements alimentaires: adaptations morphologiques et sensorielles, *Bulletins et Mémoires de la Société d'Anthropologie de Paris*, 11: 307–332.

Hladik, C.M., Robbe, B. and Pagézy, H. (1986) Differential taste thresholds among Pygmy and non Pygmy rain forest populations, Sudanese and Eskimo, with reference to the biochemical environment (in French), *Comptes Rendus de l'Académie des Sciences de Paris*, 303: 453–458.

Iaconelli, S. and Simmen, B. (1999) Palatabilité de l'acide tannique dans une solution sucrée chez *Microcebus murinus*: variation saisonnière et implication dans le comportement alimentaire, *Primatologie*, 2: 421–434.

Johansson, B., Drake, B., Pangborn, R.M., Barylko-Pikielna, N. and Koster, E.P. (1973) Difference taste thresholds for sodium chloride among young adults: an interlaboratory study, *Journal of Food Science*, 38: 524–527.

Laing, D.G., Prescott, J., Bell, G.A., Gillmore, R., James, C., Best, D.J., Allen, S., Yoshida, M. and Yamazaki, K. (1993) A cross-cultural study of taste discrimination with Australian and Japanese, *Chemical Senses*, 18: 161–168.

Likert, R. (1932) A technique for the measurement of attitudes, *Archives of Psychology*, 140: 1–55.

Looy, H. and Weingarten H.P. (1992) Facial expressions and genetic sensitivity to 6-n-propylthiouracil predict hedonic response to sweet, *Physiology and Behavior*, 52: 75–82.

Meilgaard, M., Civille, G.V. and Carr, B.T. (1987) *Sensory evaluation techniques*, CRC Press, Boca-Raton, Florida

Monneuse, M.O., Marez, A., Pasquet, P., Simmen, B. and Hladik, C.M. (2000) Sur le goût des tannins et la perception d'une substance amère (PROP), *Bulletins et Mémoires de la Société d'Anthropologie de Paris*, 12: 423–430.

Pangborn, R.M. (1959) Influence of hunger on sweetness preferences and taste thresholds, *American Journal of Clinical Nutrition*, 7: 280–287.

Pasquet, P., Oberti, B., El Ati, J. and Hladik, C.M. (2002) Relationships between threshold-based PROP sensitivity and food preferences of Tunisians, *Appetite*, 39: 167–173.

Peryam, R.D. and Pilgrim, J.F. (1957) Hedonic scale method for measuring food preferences, *Food Technology*, 11: 9–14.

Richter, C.P. and Campbell, K.H. (1939) Sucrose taste thresholds of rats and humans, *American Journal of Physiology*, 128: 291–297.

Rolls, E.T. (1997) Neural processing underlying food selection. In Macbeth, H. (ed.) *Food preferences and taste: continuity and change*, Berghahn Books, Oxford: 39–53.

Schutz, H.G. and Cardello, A.V. (2001) A labeled affective magnitude (LAM) scale for assessing food liking/disliking, *Journal of Sensory Studies*, 16: 117–159.

Simmen, B. and Hladik, C.M. (1988) Seasonal variation of taste threshold for sucrose in a prosimian species, *Microcebus murinus, Folia Primatologica,* 51: 152–157.

Simmen, B., Josseaume, B. and Atramentowicz, M. (1999) Frugivory and taste responses to fructose and tannic acid in a prosimian primate and a didelphid marsupial, *Journal of Chemical Ecology*, 25: 331–346.

Steiner, J.E. (1977) Facial expressions of the neonate infant indicating the hedonics of food-related chemical stimuli. In Weiffenbach, J.M. (ed.) *Taste and Development: epigenetic of sweet preferences*, NIH-DHEW, Bethesda: 173–189.

Steiner, J.E. and Glaser, D. (1984) Differential behavioral responses to taste stimuli in nonhuman primates, *Journal of Human Ecology*, 13: 709–723.

Whissel-Buechy, D. (1990) Effects of age and sex on taste sensitivity to phenylthiocarbamide (PTC) in the Berkeley Guidance sample, *Chemical Senses*, 15: 39–57.

# 8. RESEARCHING FOOD PREFERENCES

## METHODS AND PROBLEMS FOR ANTHROPOLOGISTS

*Helen Macbeth* and *Fiona Mowatt*

### Introduction

The study of human food preferences is indeed an area for cross-disciplinary discussion (Macbeth 1997), as biochemical processes and life experiences interrelate in the formation of each individual's preferences and aversions. On the one hand, neurophysiologists and their colleagues in physiological psychology study the neurological pathways and neuronal responses of both the gustatory and the olfactory sensations involved. Rolls (1997) wrote a simplified introduction to these biochemical processes, and their integration in the brain, for anthropologists and other non-specialists, but, as the neurological sciences are advancing at a fast rate, a prospective researcher, interested in the neurophysiology of sensory perceptions, should search the literature for the most recent material available.

On the other hand, food preferences are not only based on these biochemical processes, genetic and non-genetic in origin. Even the biochemical components are not all 'innate' but develop as they interact with both biological and social experiences throughout the course of life. Even supposedly purely biological aspects cannot be separated from culturally learned and individual psychological responses (Hladik and Simmen 1996). While these different sorts of experiences all act on the individual, it is clear that cultural factors also affect all such socialisation. These cultural factors do not just comprise differing ideas about the edible and the inedible. They also extend to differing ideas of cuisine and to differing expectations about one's behaviour, whether related to one's gender or age, or even just to the time of day or year. In European societies such expectations are most clearly demonstrated in regard to which drinks, especially alcoholic drinks, are appropriate (for examples see Garine and Garine 2001).

Food aversions, including strong physical feelings of disgust, are the opposite of food preferences. Socially and culturally induced food preferences and aversions can become unconsciously integrated in the physiological reactions of the individual (Schiefenhövel 1997), while previous biological experiences, such as a coincident sickness (see Simmen *et al.* this volume), can become part of the cognitive attitude to the foods in question. Garcia *et al.* (1968) stimulated a feeling of nausea in laboratory rats, using X-rays, and from then on the rats would not eat the food given them just before the sickness caused by the rays. Readers may know of their own family examples of this phenomenon – the marmalade containing medication before an operation is disliked for years – a new food given to a child going down with measles may be avoided for life, etc. The dislike is understood and cognitive, even if the original cause is not remembered or recognised.

Whereas research into the causes, the aetiology, of food preferences must include an understanding of all this inextricable biosocial complexity, anthropologists, nutritionists and epidemiologists have tended to be more concerned with the consequences or the social significance of the preferences, than in the preferences themselves, or their aetiology. Nevertheless, acquiring information on human differences in food preferences is relevant to these other studies, and this chapter will focus on ways to describe or compare food preferences of a group or groups of people.

Since, whatever the aetiology, individuals usually do have a concept of their own food preferences and aversions, humans can be asked about these. Successful research, of course, depends on respondents' ability to communicate their reactions to the researchers. The literature on the study of stated food preferences in sample populations exemplifies well the use of highly statistical approaches within the social sciences, particularly in social psychology. Messer (1986), an anthropologist, in her fieldwork in a Mexican town, noted the greater enjoyment of very sweet tastes there than she had observed was normal in the United States. She followed this by undertaking quantitative research and thereby found household-to-household variation in this (see also Messer this volume). Cultural differences have frequently been noted. For example, Rozin and Schiller (1980) discussed cultural differences in tastes for what we call 'hot' dishes with chilli. Even the lay public has come to expect preferences to differ between cultural groups, although the exemplification of such differences in some of the currently popular 'ethnic' cookbooks should be treated with scepticism. However, if what is thought to be exotic is also considered *chic* for dinner parties, then this too can develop into a preference despite being exotic (see James 1997). This is linked to a belief in the high status of a food frequently affecting taste preferences. In summary, the aetiology of differences in preferences for tastes and flavours, however much debated, clearly contains both biological and social elements.

It is worth noting here that preferences are not only related to gustation and olfaction, but also to feel (e.g. crunchiness) and visual image. Macbeth at a Hollowe'en party in the 1970s put harmless food dyes (blue in one pot, green in another) in the water for boiling spaghetti. Several guests would not help themselves from this dish of intertwined blue and green strands. As for the pink dyed *penne*, few felt like eating something that looked like chopped uncooked intestines or veins. Even the weird Hallowe'en naming of some very ordinary stews put some people off. The hostess had not expected this reaction to the Hallowe'en 'joke'!

Research on stated food preferences is primarily found within the discipline of social psychology, but researchers in market forces and some nutritionists have also contributed to the topic. Their studies have mostly been concerned with sectors of a single population, especially age groups. Age, gender and socioeconomic differences are regularly shown (e.g. Conner 1993, 1994). A great deal of research has been concerned with food preferences in young children (e.g. Alles-White and Welch 1985), and the majority of that material has been concerned with understanding the development of the preferences. Educationalists and anthropologists have joined the psychologists and nutritionists in the study of the food preferences of older children, adolescents and young adults. Harper's name should be mentioned for his life's work on the topic (for a review of his research see Frijters 1988). Genetic influences on preference have been investigated by testing identical and non-identical twins and asking them to rate their preferences (e.g. Falciglia and Norton 1994).

Although there is generally a close relationship between preferences and choices, in many parts of the world, poverty allows no, or almost no, choice. Perhaps to the surprise of the affluent, Garine (1997) and González Turmo (1997) each discussed that in such circumstances the poor expressed a 'preference' for the food item that they did eat, and not for some rare treat. Preferences, therefore, can only affect choices when choices exist or can be afforded, but preferences can still be expressed in the absence of choice. In contrast, it is common for more affluent people to seek variety and new experiences. As well as the cognitive aspects of this search for variety, there are also physiological reasons (Rolls 1997) for this when satiety of one food reduces one's appetite for it. Nevertheless, choice and preference are linked in other ways too. Where a food has a scarcity value, usually linked to greater expense, it may gain status among the affluent. Similar to the discussion above of what is considered *chic*, this may develop into a cognitive 'preference'. Furthermore, beliefs in the health value of foods, strongly fostered today by advertisers (Macbeth and Collinson in press), can become so fundamental to an individual that preferences are affected.

What is clear from the above is that there are many components to the development of preferences. Furthermore, the preferences may be labile, changing with other circumstances in the individual's life, socioeconomic situation, time of year, climate, time of day, satiety, health or otherwise, etc. So, any researcher wishing to study preferences should bear in mind that a response is just a response at that moment in that individual's life. The readers of this volume will already be well aware of the desirability of combining methods of research and if possible spending long enough in the research area for participant observation.

## Research Methods

### Laboratory Research

There are several methods of testing for preferences (for useful overviews, see Institute of Food Technologists 1981, MacFie and Thomson 1994). Some are laboratory based and subjects have to taste and comment on substances given to them (for simple introductions and even test templates for these, see www.nutrition.org.uk/education/teachercentre.html). The subject may be given two substances in a 'paired-preference test' and asked to state their preference between the two substances. In some cases, one of the substances is duplicated and the subject is provided with two substances but in three containers. When more than two substances are provided, the subject is asked to rank their preference for the substances. Such methods are generally known as 'ranking tests'. Sometimes subjects are asked to rate their preference for a substance or series of substances on some kind of scale. (The discussion on scales continues below.)

### Questionnaires

Self-administered questionnaires, which do not require substances or laboratories are also common in this kind of research. These can be as simple as questionnaires with *agree, not sure* and *disagree* options to statements made about the desirability of food items. However, more common are questions which require an answer along a rating scale of high to low. This can be expressed as a rating 'from 5 high to 1 low', or five options might be given, e.g. *like very much, like, indifferent, dislike, dislike very strongly*, and subjects would be asked to choose an option. These options might be typed to be encircled, as in multiple choice answers, or each option might head a column for the whole list. The former type are familiar to many of us from market research questionnaires, while in the latter case, respondents simply put a mark in the correct column. When there are only a few columns or options, this kind of research is very simple and quick to analyse, for example by chi-square analysis. Although specialist studies have progressed to more complex scaling (as discussed below), some students and new researchers should not be dissuaded from the simplicity of this approach, as it can still be useful, especially in conjunction with other methods of study (e.g. Randall and Sanjur 1981). The questionnaires can be used as part of an interview, or distributed for self-administration. They are easy to administer because they are easy to understand. However, when in combination with other forms of anthropological research they can provide some useful quantitative data.

Macbeth, Green and Castro became involved in a study of food preferences almost by chance. In the creation of a low-budget way to collect 7-day food intake frequency data (Macbeth 1995, Henry and Macbeth this volume), they only wanted to create a way to familiarise schoolchildren with filling in columns on a response form. Castro (personal communication) suggested a simple questionnaire with four columns for preferences (*like very much, like, indifferent, dislike*) and three columns for concepts about health value of the foods (*good for health to eat frequently, neither good nor bad for health, bad for health to eat frequently*). A form was designed to be a cheerful, easily understood 'game' to be 'played' in each class, but the children undertook the task seriously. We were surprised how easily we had gathered some interesting data, since the schools were in different nations. The data were swiftly coded and very simply analysed by chi-square analysis, showing many significant differences between boys and girls (Macbeth *et al.* 1990) and between French and Spanish samples (Macbeth and Green 1997). The first criticism of the above method is that options on the *like* side of neutral exceeded the one option for *dislike*. More general criticisms, however, relate to the crude simplicity of the method, a simplicity which also resulted in a benefit with the ease and speed of analysis. Macbeth was able, for example, to give the schools a brief report on the results within a couple of days, while still in the fieldwork area, considerably enhancing good will for the rest of the research. Also, the method has been used successfully in an undergraduate project. Nevertheless, it should be noted that this method may be considered too crude and unsophisticated for many research purposes (see also Medina, this volume).

## Hedonic Scales

Because the options above are ranked, they can also be considered as scales. Scales for expressing like to dislike or pleasure to displeasure have been called 'hedonic scales'. Generally it is argued that it is preferable for an uneven number of options to be used, so that there exists a central option for indifference. However, several researchers (e.g. Jones *et al.* 1955, Gridgeman 1961, Olsen 1999) draw attention to the problems in having a neutral centre point, while its absence forces respondents to make positive or negative choices. A 5-point hedonic scale is one where there are five options from strong like (5) to strong dislike (1) and, as mentioned above, was used by Randall and Sanjur (1981: 155) 'because of its known simplicity and effectiveness'.

However, by far the most frequently used of the hedonic scales is the 9-point hedonic scale (Peryam and Girardot 1952, Peryam and Pilgrim 1957). The nine options are from *like extremely* to *dislike extremely*, the central option being *neither like nor dislike*. Once the options exceed five, it is preferable that the

***Figure 8.1***  Example of a 9-point hedonic scale *(after Peryam and Pilgrim 1957)*

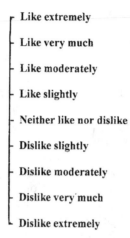

options are displayed along a graphic line, which demonstrates the idea of a scale. Such a 9-point hedonic scale (Figure 8.1) was originally designed at the United States Army Quartermaster Food and Container Institute, Chicago, and was tested on military personnel. It was quickly taken up as a research method by a wide range of other researchers, both in industry and in academic and governmental studies, and, as often happens, its frequent use became the rationale for adoption in further research. That remains the case today.

Nevertheless, there are criticisms of aspects of this 9-point hedonic scale (for example, see Simmen *et al.* this volume). The discussions are mostly based on mathematical or statistical problems in relation to the analysis of data that result from use of the scale. The reader interested in pursuing this to a higher level would find the discussion by Schutz and Cardello (2001) stimulating. This is primarily a debate about the intervals along the scale. While, in the usual 9-point hedonic scale (Figure 8.1), the options are spaced equally along the scale, Schutz and Cardello developed a 'labeled affective magnitude scale' (LAM), for which there are eleven options, because beyond *like extremely* and *dislike extremely*, they have added *greatest imaginable like* and *greatest imaginable dislike*. They wanted to offer options beyond the 'extreme' to the 'imaginable'. Furthermore, the options they proposed are clustered more closely in the centre, with a wider gap between moderate options either side and the widest gaps between *like extremely* and *greatest imaginable like* and between *dislike extremely* and *greatest imaginable dislike* (see Figure 7.5, Simmen *et al.* this volume). Essentially, this is for two reasons: firstly because in the near neutral categories the differences in preference are probably quite slight, and secondly because they wanted to create a significant gap between *extremely* and *greatest imaginable*, with the idea that the latter is almost beyond reality.

Although the options are placed unevenly along the scale, the scale itself still has regular measurements along it, whether shown or not. Subjects are asked to respond about a given food by expressing their preference as a diagonal line through the scale and where that line crosses the scale will have a numerical value which can be used for analysis. Schutz and Cardello (2001) also discuss whether the numeric values should be shown along the scale or not and whether they should be from '0' to '100' or from '–100' to '+100'.

However, what should be noted by anthropologists is that the literature in, for example, the *Journal of Sensory Studies*, about the relative values of different hedonic scales, results from studies within single populations. Other issues arise when one is involved in designing a method for comparison across two or more different cultures, as is discussed in the next section.

## Feasibility Study for Five-nation Research

The authors of this chapter were given the opportunity to design research methods for studying taste and preference for a feasibility study financed by a grant from the European Union. The situation was that methods should be designed and tested on population samples from five European nations, Belgium, France, Italy, Spain and United Kingdom We divided the components between laboratory-type research into tests on 'gustation' (Hladik *et al.* 2002, Simmen *et al.* this volume) and on recognition and assessment of odours, on the one hand, and on self-administered questionnaires on preference and attitude on the other. The tests on gustation have been discussed in the previous chapter and those on olfaction were never usefully analysed in relation to food choices. So, only those for preference and attitude are discussed below.

We found that in the cross-disciplinary literature the terms, 'preference' and 'acceptability' are not always clearly differentiated, but anthropologists will probably prefer to reserve the word 'acceptability' for description of the concepts in different cultures of what is considered 'edible'. In the wider literature, there is also use of the word, 'attitude', which we chose to interpret only as 'social attitude'. We experimented with several methods for testing people's social attitudes to certain foods, but in the end did not carry out trials of these. For one of these the subject has to associate foods with photos of stereotypes of Europeans from different age groups and different socioeconomic classifications. For another, a selection of drinks (alcoholic and non-alcoholic, hot and cold) have to be deemed appropriate, or otherwise, for each of a series of situations, both for the respondent and for each person on a list of different stereotyped categories of people. Neither of these tests are discussed further here. What we describe below is our experiences in creating methods for testing preference by questionnaires that would be easy to complete by respondents of different educational levels in different European countries.

## Hedonic Scales

We first worked on the primary principle of the 9-point hedonic scale for study-ing preferences, but we had prior information about Schutz and Cardello's LAM scale (published later in 2001) and decided to use their scaling with eleven points and a numbered scale from '–100' to '+100'. Respondents had to make a short diagonal mark through the scale at the point that reflected their concept of their preference level. However, our decisions did not end there. We had to translate the categories appropriately. It is insufficient simply to use a dictionary or a non-local translator; it is essential that help with choice of the words on the scale is given by a local, native speaker of each language. We would not be in laboratory situations and would have to design a self-admin-istered questionnaire, even if this was to be completed with an interviewer present. The instructions had to be clear, and in each language.

Next, we had to decide upon the food items to be listed for judgement. Here, there can be conflict between what is ideal for the topic in question and what one can reasonably expect the respondent to tolerate without losing interest. Our research topic related to so-called 'Mediterranean foods' and at first we wanted to include both 'Southern' and 'Northern' European foods for con-trast. However, there were constraints imposed on us to include some specific 'Mediterranean foods' and most of the 'Northern' food items had in the end to be dropped. The new researcher must always take into serious consideration the tolerance of the subject for spending time on any one research activity. We decided upon thirty-six items, but as the research trial continued, we had to add three more.

Translation of these food words, too, required careful discussion with native speakers. There are many unforeseen complications here; as one example the words for sweet and hot peppers had to be distinguished. Another example is that we had included *garlic* as an item. We had worked out that we should have both *cooked garlic* and *raw garlic*. However, Macbeth was surprised to find that nearly all in the trial in a small village in southern Italy responded with dislike for *cooked garlic*. It turned out that they disliked finding whole cooked cloves of garlic in dishes, and so a further alternative of *crushed garlic in sauces, etc.* was added (see also Macbeth *et al.* 1999). Other problems arose – should *cabbage* be listed as cooked or raw? – in fact should one make any comments about cuisine? – should one try to find equivalent local names for the mild and the strong cheeses, etc.? The new researcher should bear all such problems in mind, especially when undertaking cross-cultural study.

Once the scale and the food items had been chosen, we had to consider the layout of the questionnaire. The easiest to reproduce would be a single page, with the scale repeated horizontally on each row beside a different food item, but this has the problem described as 'tracking' when the respondent has a ten-dency to be influenced by where they had marked the scale above (Pasquet personal communication). With this in mind, we decided that each food item and scale should be printed on its own strip and that the strips should be

*Figure 8.2*  Example of a 'strip' with 11-point hedonic scale used in five-nation trials

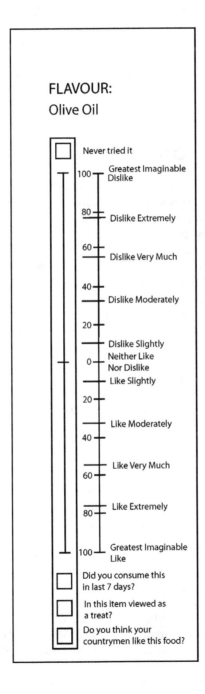

stapled together in little narrow booklets. Once we had this pattern in mind, like many researchers we could not resist asking just a little more information about frequency and attitude (Figure 8.2) and three more questions were added to each page. However, having administered these questionnaires in several countries under quite different conditions, Macbeth warns against this temptation to add in just a little more information. The three little questions, although simple to answer, were disruptive to the flow and took time that could have been spent on further food items. Nevertheless, researchers can make their own decisions about this.

## Scales for Views on Other Perspectives

As discussed above in our introduction, other aspects of choice become closely interrelated with preferences, and we chose to create similar little booklets of scales for concepts about the healthiness of each food item and about the cost of items. As we were no longer dealing with hedonic scales, we abandoned the Schutz and Cardello LAM type of scaling but retained eleven options, including the *imaginable* options at either end. We put the options evenly along the scales, still numbered from '–100' to '+100' (Figures 8.3 and 8.4). For several reasons the food items chosen could not always be the same as in the preferences booklets; for example, garlic is only bought in its raw state. However, there was a certain level of concordance between booklets where viable.

## Putting the Study Together

Finally, different coloured paper was used for each of the booklets, so that for all nations, yellow was used for the preferences booklets, orange for health beliefs and grey for costs. Furthermore, each booklet had three pages with the appropriate scale on but no food item. These proved to be very useful when the experience of the pilot studies led us to add items. We also inserted into the white instruction 'cover' sheet, questions on age, gender, occupation and country and region of birth. We of course knew current residence. For an example of use of the above method see Pasquet *et al.* (2002).

Armed now with the white cover sheet and three different coloured booklets for each subject, in different languages but comparable, we next had to study our interviewing techniques in different settings and different nations. We had to estimate timing per individual and how to be as efficient as possible both of researcher time and of respondent's patience. This method is well suited to house visits, when several family members can be given the booklets during one visit, when other aspects of a household study could also be carried out if wished. However, we were able to demonstrate that, given the right circumstances, we could achieve a cheerful atmosphere and a very efficient turn-around of respondents by holding a well organised timetable of visits in one

**Figure 8.3** Example of a 'strip' with 11-point scale for concept of health value

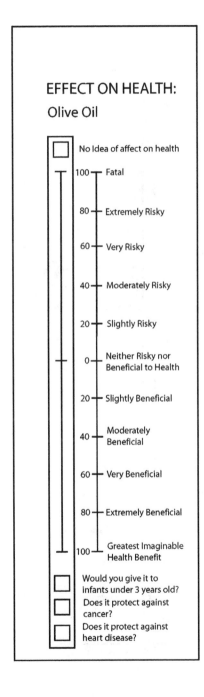

***Figure 8.4***   Example of a 'strip' with 11-point scale for concept of cost

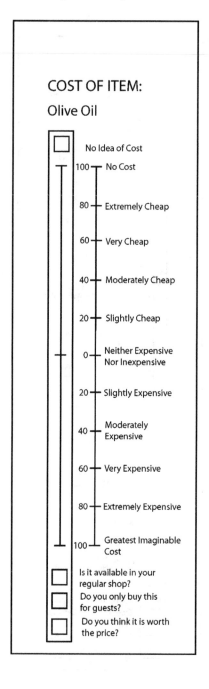

local place, for example, as in one small town in Belgium, the health centre. Under such circumstances the method approximates a more 'laboratory' approach. Such efficiency achieves more data more quickly and more cheaply, but much information is lost in comparison with a home visit and probable relaxed chat over a cup of coffee.

## Statistical Analysis

Data entry can be easily carried out in Excel or in the data entry program of any statistical package. In our study, subjects were given a serial number based on locality of current residence to avoid use of any names. The information on the cover sheets was transformed to codes and entered on to the computer. The information on the coloured booklets was very easy to code, as each diagonal line through a scale represented a number between –100 and +100 on that scale. The three extra questions also were easy code with 1 for 'yes', 2 for 'no' and something for blank. When these data were added, each 'case' was completed on a computer 'file' ready for statistical analysis. As mentioned in other chapters, we do not feel that this book should contain discussions of the advantages

*Figure 8.5*  Example of results from five-nation trials, displaying differences in hedonic scale scores by boxplot graphs: national diversity regarding preference for olive oil

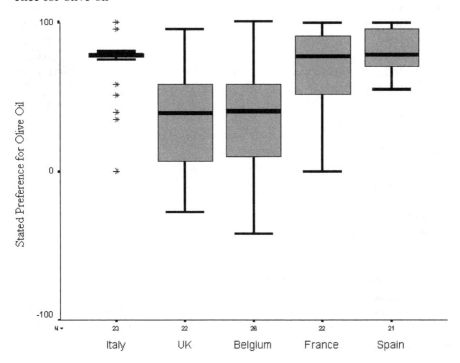

and disadvantages of different statistical methods, but the first task is always to look for the 'normality' of distribution curves. Then we used analysis of variance to compare different national samples and found many significant differences. Figure 8.5 shows how differences can be displayed by box plots.

We used Student Newman Keul tests to show how, in the results, some nations clustered more closely together than other nations. We also used factorial analysis and then studied how the resultant 'factors' broke down by nation, sex and age, and again how the nations 'clustered'. Where food items corresponded sufficiently well across the different coloured booklets, it was of interest to see how these correlated with each other. These few comments are sufficient to show that these data allow opportunities for a variety of statistical analyses, but unless the distributions are shown to be 'normal', the researcher is reminded to use nonparametric methods.

## Conclusion

After introducing methods for testing preferences, which can be studied from other sources, this chapter has provided the reader with an example of the issues one comes across when designing quantitative methods for research into food preferences and attitudes across different cultural groups. We emphasised the problems involved in finding the correct translations of words. However, there are more differences than just the words, for there are cultural interpretations of those words. Such differences occur not only in how the food item is presumed to be prepared (or in the questions asked about which preparation one is considering), but also in the interpretation of the scales. In some cultures, it may be more acceptable to be moderate in all responses, while in other cultures the extreme categories are expressed more readily. The limitation of the elegant mathematical discussions about scales (e.g. Schutz and Cardello 2001, Villanueva et al. 2002) is that they were used for research each within one population. However, cultural differences in the perception of a scale were shown by Yeh et al. (1998) in their research comparing responses between Americans, Chinese, Koreans and Thai.

Our conclusion, therefore, is that one cannot assume that any scaling will be used consistently across different cultures, or even across different socioeconomic, gender or age groups apparently sharing the same culture, and the researcher should be aware of this. If the prime researcher(s) take the time to be involved in administering questionnaires themselves, or at least in carrying out the pilot study, they will observe reactions to the scales. The point is that if reactions to these scales are very different between cultural groups, e.g. with significantly different ranges of variances, then the mathematical advantages of the more complex scales, whether traditional 9-point or LAM or other, over the simple five option rankings mentioned earlier may be lost. As in other chapters in this volume, the authors strongly recommend that researchers undertaking research into food habits involve themselves in more than one research method, whether for studying one population or for comparing populations, and that they should spend some time in participant observation.

## Acknowledgements

The authors wish to thank all those in Belgium, France, Italy, Spain and United Kingdom on whom the international trials were carried out. We also want to thank all the assistants who helped us with these trials, in particular Francesco Grippo (who also helped with the analysis), Catherine Burnotte and Marie-Hélène Avalonne, who carried out some of the trials in the authors' absence. Finally, the European grant CCE DG V/SOC97 200420 05F02 is acknowledged, although never totally received. The coordination of the European feasibility project (COMER No97/CAN/45916) was by Mariette Gerber and Martine Padilla, and we are grateful for constructive comments from *all* the international team involved, particularly for the comments by Patrick Pasquet. In regard to the work in the Cerdanya valley, ESRC grant no. R-000-232816 is acknowledged, and the local schools, teenagers and all participants thanked.

## References

Alles-White, M.L. and Welch, P. (1985) Factors affecting the formation of food preferences in pre-school children, *Early Child Development and Care*, 21: 265–76.

Conner, M.T. (1993) Individualized measurement of attitudes towards food, *Appetite*, 20(3): 235–238.

Conner, M.T. (1994) Accounting for gender, age and socioeconomic differences in food choice, *Appetite*, 23: 195.

Falciglia, G.A. and Norton, P.A. (1994) Evidence for a genetic influence on preference for some foods, *Journal of American Dietetic Association*, 94(2): 154–158.

Frijters, J.E.R. (1988) A review of Roland Harper's research in psychology and food science. In Thompson, D.M.H. (ed.) *Food Acceptability*, Elsevier Science, London: 11–25.

Garcia, J., McGowan, B.K., Ervin, F.R. and Koelling, R.A. (1968) Cues: their relative effectiveness as a function of the reinforcer, *Science*, 169: 794–795 [cited in Schiefenhövel 1997].

Garine, I. de (1997) Food preferences and taste in an African perspective: a word of caution. In Macbeth, H. (ed.) *Food Preferences and Taste: continuity and change*, Berghahn, Oxford:187–207.

Garine, I. de and Garine, V. de (2001) *Drinking: anthropological approaches*, Berghahn, Oxford.

González Turmo, I. (1997) The pathways of taste: the west Andalucian case. In Macbeth, H. (ed.) *Food Preferences and Taste: continuity and change*, Berghahn, Oxford: 115–126.

Gridgeman, N.T. (1961) A comparison of some taste-test methods, *Journal of Food Science*, 26: 171–177 [cited in Schutz and Cardello 2001].

Hladik, C.M. and Simmen, B. (1996) Taste perception and feeding behavior in non-human primates and human populations, *Evolutionary Anthropology*, 5: 58–71.

Institute of Food Technologists (1981) *Sensory Evaluation Guide for Testing Food and Beverage Produce*, Sensory Evaluation Division, Institute of Food Technologists, Chicago.

James, A.C. (1997) How British is British food? A view from anthropology. In Caplan, P. (ed.) *Food, Identity and Health*, Routledge, London: 71–86.

Jones, I.V., Peryam, D.R. and Thurstone, L.L. (1955) Development of a scale for measuring soldiers' food preference, *Food Research*, 20: 512–520.

Macbeth, H. (1995) The Cerdanya, a valley divided: biosocial anthropology in a research project. In Boyce, A.J. and Reynolds, V. (eds) *Human Populations: diversity and adaptation*, Oxford University Press, Oxford: 233–251.

Macbeth, H. (1997) (ed.) *Food Preferences and Taste: continuity and change,* Berghahn, Oxford.

Macbeth, H. and Collinson, P. (in press), Are beliefs in 'Science' rational? Concepts about healthy foods. In Millán, A., Cantarero, L., Medina, F.X. and Portalatín, M.J. (eds) *Arbitrario cultural y alimentación: racionalidad e irracionalidad del comportamento alimentario; homenaje al Dr. Igor de Garine*, Diputación Provincial de Zaragoza, Zaragoza.

Macbeth, H. and Green, A. (1997) Nationality and food preferences in the Cerdanya valley, eastern Pyrenees. In Macbeth, H. (ed.) *Food Preferences and Taste: continuity and change*, Berghahn, Oxford: 139–154.

Macbeth, H., Green, A. and Castro, A. (1990) Gender differences in adolescent views about food: a study of teenage food preferences in a Pyrenean valley, *Social Biology and Human Affairs*, 55(2): 79–92.

Macbeth, H., Grippo, F. and Roberts, D. (1999) Garlic surprise: unexpected quantitative results explained by a more qualitative approach, *Social Biology and Human Affairs*, 64(2): 14–21.

MacFie, H.J.H. and Thomson, D.M.H. (1994) (eds) *Measurement of Food Preferences*, Chapman and Hall, London.

Messer, E. (1986) Some like it sweet: estimating sweetness preferences and sucrose intakes from ethnographic and experimental data, *American Anthropologist*, 88: 637–647.

Olsen, S.O. (1999) Strength and conflicting valence in the measurement of food attitude preferences, *Food Quality and Preference*, 10(6): 483–494 [cited in Schutz and Cardello 2001].

Pasquet, P., Oberti, B., El Ati, J. and Hladik, C.M. (2002) Relationships between the threshold-based PROP sensitivity and food preferences of Tunisians, *Appetite*, 39: 167–173.

Peryam, D.R. and Girardot, N.F. (1952) Advanced taste-test method, *Journal of Food engineering*, 24: 58–61.

Peryam, D.R. and Pilgrim, F.J. (1957) Hedonic scale method of measuring food preference, *Food Technology*, 11: 9–14.

Randall, E. and Sanjur, D. (1981) Food preferences – their conceptualization and relationship to consumption, *Ecology of Food and Nutrition*, 11: 151–161.

Rolls, E.T. (1997) Neural processing underlying food selection. In Macbeth, H. (ed.) *Food Preferences and Taste: continuity and change,* Berghahn, Oxford: 39–54.

Rozin, P. and Schiller, D. (1980) The nature and acquisition of a preference for chilli pepper by humans, *Motivation and Emotion*, 4: 77–101.

Schiefenhövel, W. (1997) Good taste and bad taste: preferences and aversions as biological principles. In Macbeth, H. (ed.) *Food Preferences and Taste: continuity and change,* Berghahn, Oxford: 55–64.

Schutz, H.G. and Cardello, A.V. (2001) A labeled affective magnitude (LAM) scale for assessing food liking/disliking, *Journal of Sensory Studies*, 16: 117–159.

Villanueva, N.D.M., Da Silva, M.A.A.P. and Petenate, A.J. (2002) Performance of the self-adjusting and hybrid hedonic scales in the generation of Internal Preference Maps [paper given at the Annual Meeting and Food Expo – Anaheim, California], (ift.confex.com/ift2002/techprogram/paper_13714.htm)

Yeh, L.L., Kim, K.O., Chompreeda, P., Rimkeeree, H., Yau, N.J.N., Lundahl, D.S. (1998) Comparison in use of the 9-point hedonic scale between Americans, Chinese, Koreans and Thai, *Food Quality and Preference*, 9(6): 413–419.

www.nutrition.org.uk/education/teachercentre.html

# 9. DIETARY INTAKE METHODS IN THE ANTHROPOLOGY OF FOOD AND NUTRITION

*Stanley J. Ulijaszek*

Dietary and nutritional studies in anthropology may attempt to address issues in which food and nutrition are central, or where diet may be a peripheral or contributory component of a complex of problems within a group, population or society. Studies may be directly concerned with nutritional factors or they may be concerned with food symbolism, the perception of food, or the role of food in forging and maintaining identity. Dietary intake studies can be used to inform the study of food consumption, nutrient intake and nutritional status. Thus the range of ways that dietary intake studies can serve anthropological enquiry is extremely broad. The choice of method or methods should involve the degree of appropriateness for the question in hand, the accuracy, precision, complexity, and cost (in time and money) of the techniques chosen, and the ease of subsequent interpretation of quantitative results. This is often not straightforward, and the aim of this chapter is to examine critically some of the problems associated with the choice and use of dietary methods in determining food and nutrient intake, and in estimating nutritional status from nutrient intake. Various books have been written about measurement of diet and nutritional intake, and nutritional status assessment from dietary intakes. Most of them consider the role of dietary and nutritional factors in human health. Volumes considering the study of diet and nutrition in anthropology include those edited by Johnston (1987) and Pelto *et al.* (1989) and written by Ulijaszek and Strickland (1993). Readers wanting more information than is possible to give in the present chapter are guided to these volumes.

## Food, Nutrients and Nutritional Status

Dietary studies carried out by anthropologists can be divided into three main types: those concerned directly with food consumption; those concerned with nutrient, including energy, intake; and those concerned with nutritional status. The quantitative study of food and nutrition has three levels of methodological application (Table 9.1). First, the study of diet needs some measure of different types of food eaten across a given time frame. The estimate of food eaten may be either retrospective, concurrent or prospective, and may involve observations of the frequencies of consumption of different foods, or the actual amounts eaten. The study of nutrient intakes requires the measurement of quantities of different foods eaten, which can then be converted into amounts of nutrients eaten by the application of food composition table values. Nutrients are chemical compounds found in food, which are essential for some aspect or aspects of bodily function. Quantitatively, dietary energy needs (which come from the macronutrients carbohydrate, protein and fat) are the most important, since they control physiological hunger. Hunger is appeased when these energy needs are met. In this context, energy is considered to be a nutrient, even though it can be provided by any mix of the three macronutrients. Protein has distinct physiological functions in the body, and is considered a nutrient in its own right. Some fats have beneficial effects for human physiology, and are also considered to be nutrients, beyond their ability to provide dietary energy. In addition to the macronutrients, the micronutrients are nutrients that are required in small quantity. These fall into two categories, vitamins and trace elements (or minerals). The vitamins fall into two categories, fat-soluble and water-soluble. Quantitatively and functionally the most important of the fat-soluble vitamins are vitamins A, D, E and K. The most important of the water-soluble vitamins are vitamins B [$B_1$ (thiamin), $B_2$ (riboflavin), $B_3$ (niacin), $B_6$ (pyridoxin), folic acid and $B_{12}$]. The most important of the trace elements are calcium, iron, phosphorus, zinc and iodine.

The study of nutritional status from dietary intake incorporates the two steps of estimation described for the measurement of nutrient intake, as well

***Table 9.1*** Levels of estimation in dietary and nutritional studies

| | |
|---|---|
| Diet | Food intake methods |
| Nutrients | Food intake methods +<br>Conversion of foods intakes into nutrients using food composition tables |
| Nutritional status | Food intake methods +<br>Conversion of foods intakes into nutrients using food composition tables +<br>Relating nutrient intakes to recommended daily allowances |

as an additional step of estimation, which is the comparison of nutrient intakes with recommended nutrient allowances or intakes. There are different errors associated with each level of estimation, such that studies using one level of estimation (food and dietary intake) have less error associated with them than studies using two levels of estimation (nutrient intakes). Studies using three levels of estimation (nutritional status from nutrient intakes) have even more error associated with them.

## Food Intake

There are four basic approaches to the measurement of diet: the use of diet records, diet recall, diet history and food frequency questionnaire, respectively (see for example Cameron and van Staveren 1988). The more commonly used among these methods are summarised in Table 9.2. There is no single, ideal method for estimating dietary intake (Gibson 1990) and there is no merit in using a more elaborate or expensive technique than is needed for the purposes of the study (see for example Henry and Macbeth this volume). A broad generalisation is that the more detailed the desired data, the more time consuming and expensive is the method needed (Ferro-Luzzi 1982).

Furthermore, the more invasive the method, the more likely it is that the dietary intake (or the reporting thereof) would be modified from habitual patterns. It is important to identify methods that are appropriate for the level of accuracy and precision needed and to minimise subject fatigue. A number of books review critically the operational details of different dietary intake methods (Gibson 1990, Willett 1990, Margetts and Nelson 1997) and those interested should consult these documents. Another serious consideration is the possibility of under-reporting of food intake, leading to underestimates of nutrient intake, where these are also to be measured (see below). Evidence of this has been cited in a number of studies (Livingstone *et al.* 1990, Mertz *et al.* 1991, Ulijaszek 1992a).

## Nutrient Intake Studies

If a dietary intake study is sufficiently detailed, it may be possible to quantify nutrient intake from it. However, the conversion of diet into nutrient intake introduces further error, because the nutrient composition of many food items is variable, incomplete, or simply not analysed. Thus, great care is needed in the use of food composition tables; an excellent critique of their use is given by West and van Staveren (1997). There are many food composition compilations available for use in many countries and regions. Extensive lists of these can be obtained by consulting the *International Food Composition Tables Directory* (www.fao.org/infoods/) or the *Inventory of European Food Composition Databases and Tables* (food.ethz.ch/cost99/db-inventory.htm). However,

***Table 9.2.***  Dietary intake methods (from Gibson 1990)

| Method and Procedures | Uses and limitations |
| --- | --- |
| **Twenty-four-hour Recall.** Subject or caretaker recalls food intake of previous twenty-four hours in an interview. Quantities estimated in household measures using food models as memory aids and/ or to assist in quantifying portion sizes. Nutrient intakes calculated using food composition data. | Useful for assessing average *usual* intakes of a large population, provided that the sample is truly representative and that the days of the week are adequately represented. Used for international comparisons of relationship of nutrient intakes to health and susceptibility to chronic disease. Inexpensive, easy, quick, with low respondent burden so that compliance is high. Large coverage possible: can be used with illiterate individuals. Element of surprise so less likely to modify eating pattern. Single twenty-four-hour recalls likely to omit foods consumed infrequently. Relies on memory and hence unsatisfactory for the elderly and young children. Multiple replicate twenty-four-hour recalls used to estimate *usual* intakes of individuals. |
| **Estimated Food Record.** Record of all food and beverages as eaten (including snacks), over periods from one to seven days. Quantities estimated in household measures. Nutrient intakes calculated using food composition data. | Used to assess *actual* or *usual* intakes of individuals, depending on number of measurement days. Data on *usual* intakes used for diet counselling and statistical analysis involving correlation and regression. Accuracy depends on conscientiousness of subject and ability to estimate quantities. Longer time frames result in a higher respondent burden and a lower co-operation. Subjects must be literate. |
| **Weighed Food Record.** All food consumed over defined period is weighed by the subject, caretaker, or assistant. Food samples may be saved individually, or as a composite, for nutrient analysis. Alternatively, nutrient intakes calculated from food composition data. | Used to assess *actual* or *usual* intakes of individuals, depending on the number of measurement days. Accurate but time consuming. Condition must allow weighing. Subjects may change their usual eating pattern to simplify weighing or to impress investigator. Requires literate, motivated, and willing participants. Expensive. |
| **Dietary History.** Interview method consisting of a twenty-four-hour recall of *actual* intake, plus information on overall *usual* eating pattern, followed by a food frequency questionnaire to verify and clarify initial data. Usual portion sizes recorded in household measures. Nutrient intakes calculated using food composition data. | Used to describe *usual* food and/or nutrient intakes over a relatively long time period which can be used to estimate prevalence of inadequate intakes. Such information used for national food policy development, food fortification planning, and to identify food patterns associated with inadequate intakes. Labour intensive, time consuming and results depend on skill of interviewer. |
| **Food Frequency Questionnaire.** Uses comprehensive list or list of specific food items to record intakes over a given period (day, week, month, year). Record is obtained by interview, or self-administered questionnaire. Questionnaire can be semi-quantitative when subjects asked to quantify usual portion sizes of food items, with or without the use of food models | Designed to obtain qualitative, descriptive data on *usual* intakes of foods or classes of foods over a long time period. Useful in epidemiological studies for ranking subjects into broad categories of low, medium and high intakes of specific foods, food components or nutrients, for comparison with the prevalence and/or mortality statistics of a specific disease. Can also identify food patterns associated with inadequate intakes of specific nutrients. Method is rapid with low respondent burden and high response rate but accuracy is lower than other methods. |

very few of these lists give variability around the reported mean values (West and van Staveren 1997). Such data would be valuable in determining errors in estimates of nutrient intake, which might be caused by variability in the nutrient content of the reference foods given in the food composition tables. Food composition tables also rarely give a complete coverage of all the foods likely to be used by a group or population. This is because the majority of intake of most nutrients is usually provided by a relatively small number of foods and compilers of the food composition tables focus their resources on these foods. It is important to assign values to all foods reported as consumed, since omission would lead to underestimation. When published values are not available in the food composition table of choice, nutrient content can be assigned by using values of similar foods given in that table, by using values for that food from a different food composition table, or by giving that food the average composition of the rest of the diet. This last option is the least preferred, although it is sometimes the only option.

Food preparation techniques can affect the nutrient content of foods eaten. Furthermore, the under-recording of substances which the subject may not regard as food but which contain nutrients can result in errors of estimation. In particular, alcoholic beverages contain energy; subjects omitting to report even small amounts of alcoholic drink may have their energy intakes significantly under-reported. Another example is the use of betel-nut as a stimulant. Slaked lime (calcium hydroxide) is needed to liberate the narcotic from the nut and is frequently chewed with the nut. Swallowing only small amounts of this lime in the course of chewing can contribute substantial quantities of calcium to intake; this could easily be missed by the dietary recorder. Furthermore, habituated betel-nut chewers may swallow the chewed substance, contributing to protein intake. In studies where trace element intakes are of interest, the consumption of substantial quantities of water, in one form or another, could make important contributions.

The water content of the food can also influence the calculated nutrient content of the diet in other ways. A gross difference in water content between that of the consumed food and that of the published value used to calculate the nutrient intake may lead to enormous inaccuracies in estimated nutrient intakes. In groups where the vast majority of the energy intake is supplied by a single staple food, estimation of the water content of samples of this food allows corrections to be made to literature values prior to use in analysis. Such corrections are likely to give considerable improvements in the estimations of intake of most nutrients.

## Nutritional Status from Nutrient Intake

It is possible to make some estimates of nutritional state of individuals in specified groups by comparing actual nutrient intakes with recommended nutrient intakes. Nutrient requirements differ by age, body size and by physiological condition (for example, pregnancy and lactation) and recommendations vary among countries and according to the scientific knowledge accepted and used to underpin these recommendations. Interpretations of such scientific data and recommendations vary according to national understanding of how nutritional well-being can best be achieved in the population. They also vary in the criteria used to define dietary adequacy. In general, recommended nutrient intakes represent the average amount of a nutrient that should be obtained *per capita* in a population, if the needs of practically all members of the group are to be met. While recommendations vary, many of the underlying principles are similar. Nutrient requirements are always set for a particular group of individuals with specified characteristics, consuming a specified diet. They refer to the average nutrient need over a reasonable period of time, although what is a reasonable period of time is rarely defined. Values are usually expressed as daily requirements, although in many agricultural societies, nutrient intakes may only average out across the year, because of the seasonality of the subsistence cycle. Recommended nutrient intakes are also estimated to be levels of intake which are needed to maintain health in already healthy people; they do not allow for illness or stress. They are based on the typical dietary pattern of people in a particular country and may not be appropriate for persons following an atypical diet. This issue is problematic in countries where there is great regional variation or ethnic difference in diet. Recommended intakes are also calculated ignoring interactions between nutrients and other dietary components, because they are difficult or impossible to quantify.

Recommended nutrient intakes represent population safety-net values for most nutrients, but one exception is the recommendation for energy, where surplus intake can lead to obesity. Statistical construction includes a margin of error (usually the mean physiological value plus two standard deviations). The mean physiological value is usually the amount of nutrient needed per day to balance out daily use or losses of that nutrient. For the intake of most nutrients this margin or error allows for within-population variation in nutrient requirements for most nutrients apart from energy.

Evaluation of the nutritional state of groups can be undertaken in several ways. Mean nutrient intake can be expressed as a percentage of the recommended nutrient intake. However, this does not assess the distribution of intakes among individuals and hence the proportion of very low or very high intakes within the group. One way to take into account the distribution of intakes within a group is to examine the proportion of subjects that fall below the recommended nutrient intake. However, this does not give any estimate of intake relative to individual physiological requirement, because the recommended intake is generally the mean requirement plus two standard deviations. As a result, the nutrient requirements of some individuals will always be below the recommended nutrient intake level (Gibson 1990). Furthermore, the proportion of subjects with intakes below the recommended nutrient intake will vary according to the dietary method used, especially with respect to the number of days of intake observed: daily nutrient intakes averaged from multi-day surveys give lower variance than single-day surveys, because the averaging procedure of the former results in regression to the mean of extreme daily values.

A further possibility is to express the nutrient status of a group as a proportion of subjects with intakes below an arbitrary proportion of the recommended nutrient intake. While it might make sense simply to strip off the 'plus two standard deviations' from the recommended values, the standard deviation values are often not published along side the recommendations. Thus, a manipulation using two thirds of the recommended value, or seventy or eighty percent of it, can be used. However, there is no scientifically defined rationale for the use of any such cut-off value and while the tendency to overestimate the prevalence of inadequate nutrient intake in the group is reduced, an unknown extent of misclassification of nutrient intake status takes place. This is clearly unsatisfactory. Another approach is to use probabilities in evaluating nutrient intakes relative to recommended nutrient intakes. This gives the probability that an individual within a group does not meet either the physiological requirement, or the recommended nutrient intake and it assumes that the distribution of nutrient requirements is Gaussian (which is unknown). When assessing energy intakes (see Henry and Macbeth this volume), the intake of an individual in terms of the distribution of requirements should be used, because no margin of safety is added to the physiological requirement when the recommended energy intake is derived. When assessing intakes of all nutrients, for which two standard deviations are added to the mean as a margin of safety, the intake of individuals expressed as percentage of recommended nutrient intake should be used.

## Period of Observation

The number of days of dietary record needed to obtain an assessment of nutrient intake for a group varies with the desired level of accuracy, within- and between- subject variation in day-to-day intake and the number of subjects observed (Ferro-Luzzi 1982). In any study, a balance must be sought between different aims:

- to maximise accuracy and/or precision,
- to obtain the largest sample possible often in small communities and
- to keep the number of days of observation low, in order not to antagonise the subjects.

Various authors have examined between- and within-subject variation in energy intake, in attempts to calculate the number of days necessary to estimate valid intakes (Willett *et al.* 1985, Nelson *et al.* 1989, Black 2001) by different methods. The number of days of dietary record needed to obtain an assessment of nutrient intake for an individual depends on the intrasubject

*Figure 9.1* Nomogram to calculate the number of days of diet records required to estimate nutrient intake of an individual, at a given level of precision (from Black 1986)

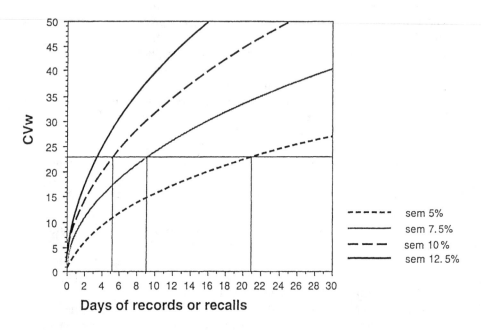

**Days of records or recalls**

coefficient of variation in daily nutrient intake (CVw) and the precision of the measurement. Figure 9.1 is a nomogram to calculate the number of days of diet records needed to estimate the nutrient intake of an individual at a given level of precision.

The determination of the number of days of observations needed for a given level of precision for groups of individuals is more complex and cannot be reduced to a nomogram. This is because the number of days of dietary record needed to obtain an assessment of nutrient intake for a group varies with the desired level of accuracy, within- and between-subject variation in day-to-day intake and the number of subjects observed. The relationship can be expressed in the following manner:

$$D = 1 \times \frac{(CVw)}{4 \times (n \times (DV)) - (4 \times (CVb))}$$

where:   D = the number of days needed per person

DV = the percentage deviation from the mean nutrient intakes of the group over the period of observation

CVw = the observed within-subject coefficient of variation

CVb = the observed between-subject coefficient of variation

n = the number studied

It is possible to set DV at a number of levels, although the lower the value, the more accurate are the reported data. While a DV of 5 percent might be desirable, it may not be possible to have this level of precision. Usually, DV is set at some point between 5 and 12.5 percent.

Operating within these constraints, researchers should arrive at their own estimates of anticipated precision. These are of value in interpretation, and should be part of routine reporting of nutrient intake data. As with other research in the human sciences, there are other considerations, such as the sampling method and the need to disaggregate the data by age and sex. An excellent account of the relationships between statistical power, sampling and sample size, which need to be considered prior to any study of diet or nutrient intake, is given by Cole (1997).

Furthermore, North American women have been shown to vary their energy intakes across the menstrual cycle (Lissner et al. 1988, Tarasuk and Beaton 1991). In Papua New Guinea, Ningerum horticulturalists show no variation in intake, but enormous differences in the sources of dietary energy across seasons (Ulijaszek 1992b). Mixed horticulturalists in Chad and Cameroon (de Garine and Koppert 1990) and agriculturalists in the Gambia (Fox 1953) engage in varying levels of post-harvest gorging. Such situations should be borne in mind when considering the period of observation. Without carrying out prior investigations, it is often difficult to determine the most appropriate sampling period and protocol. There are various ways of arriving at some approximation of this, however. Ethnographic, social and nutritional literature may give some clues to variation in dietary patterns; alternatively, researchers and government officials who have worked with the population of interest may be able to provide important information. Work patterns may give an idea of day-to-day variation and seasonality in food intake may be indicated by climatic data.

## Error, Accuracy and Precision

As already mentioned, it is also important to bear in mind the likelihood of error in any of the above. Measurement error has two different components: accuracy (or validity) and precision (or repeatability, reproducibility, reliability). These concepts are illustrated in Figure 9.2. A study is considered accurate if the observations are a reasonable representation of the true situation (Margetts and Nelson 1997). This vague definition creates problems from the outset, since what is reasonable cannot be defined and there is no 'gold standard' method for the assessment of food and nutrient intake. Inaccuracy can,

***Figure 9.2***   Visual definition of accuracy (validity) and precision
(repeatability) (from Black 1999)

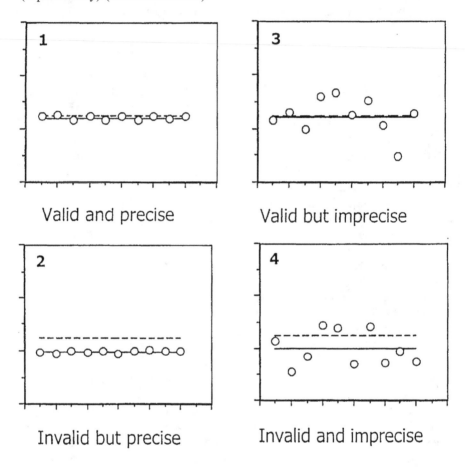

Valid and precise                    Valid but imprecise

Invalid but precise                  Invalid and imprecise

among other things, be systematic bias and may be due to instrument error, or
to errors of observation or measurement technique. Precision is the extent to
which the method used gives the same answer on repeated applications (Black
2001). Imprecision is the opposite of precision and is the variability of repeated
measurements.

The problem of a lack of adequate reference values against which to determine the accuracy of dietary records has been addressed by a number of
authors. There are various approaches which can improve the accuracy of
observations, falling into two categories. The first of these is the comparison
of energy intake with expenditure (see also Pasquet, this volume), to eliminate
low values for dietary intake. The second is the use of biomarkers against
which nutrient intake values can be compared. A list of biomarkers is given in
Table 9.3.

***Table 9.3.*** Biochemical markers or indices of nutrient intake
(From Bates and Thurnham 1997)

| Compartment | Nutrients | Comments |
|---|---|---|
| **Short term indices** | | |
| Faeces | Inorganic ions<br>Lipids | Balance studies only; for lipids one needs to consider endogenous production and contributions of colonic bacteria |
| Urine | B-vitamins [not folate or $B_{12}$], Vitamin C | Greatest variation and therefore predictive power at moderate-to-high intakes |
| | $Na^+$, $K^+$, ($Ca^{2+}$, $Mg^{2+}$)<br>Halides, sulphate, selenium | |
| | Nitrogen, urea, creatinine, 3-methyl histidine, sulphur amino acids | All require complete collections, adequate days for desired precision |
| Bile salts | Cholesterol | Metabolic ward study only |
| Breath | Fibre (hydrogen, methane) | Validity uncertain |
| Serum/plasma | All vitamins, but mainly used for vitamin $B_6$ (pyridoxal phosphate), vitamin C and the fat-soluble vitamins | Intake range for predictive power varies between nutrients, e.g. wide for water-soluble vitamins, narrow for vitamin A |
| | Some inorganic nutrients | Variable predictive power between nutrients |
| | Cholesterol, cholesteryl esters, phospholipids, triglycerides, free fatty acids | May be affected by recent diet (TG, FFA). Total FA can be me asured, better analysed in subfractions separately |
| **Medium/long term indices** | | |
| Red cells | Vitamins $B_1$, $B_2$, $B_6$<br>$B_1$, $B_6$, niacin, folate<br>Se<br>$Cu^{2+}$<br>Fatty Acids | Enzyme activation indices<br>Total co-factor concentration<br>Glutathione peroxidase<br>Superoxide dismutase |
| White cells | Vitamin C<br>Zn, Se<br>Fatty Acids | Entire 'buffy coat' generally used; separated cell types probably better Monocytes; may be only short term indicator |
| Hair, toe-nails finger-nails | (Zn, Cu and other 'trace' elements) | Controversial interpretation |
| Cheek cells | Phospholipid fatty acids | Validity uncertain |
| Adipose tissue | Fatty acids | Useful in metabolic and experimental studies |

A further way in which accuracy (or validity) can be estimated is to compare one dietary method against another. Since there is no reference value for dietary intake, this approach must be considered 'pseudovalidation' rather than validation. Usually, Pearson correlations are used in such studies and values vary enormously. Recommendations have been published for the design of validation studies for use in epidemiology, and these are summarised in Table 9.4. As discussed above the objectives in Anthropology vary greatly, but in common with epidemiology the focus is usually on groups(s) or populations.

## The use of Biomarkers

Although biochemical markers give important yardsticks for the validation of dietary intakes, they are not perfect 'gold standards'. This is because:

- The relationships between physiological factors, such as intestinal mucosal transport rates, tissue and renal threshold saturation rates, and feedback control of absorption, do not give constant relationships between the nutrient in the food eaten and the presentation of that nutrient or a metabolite of it, in particular bodily tissues.
- There is variation in the fundamental bioavailability of different chemical forms of nutrients as found in foods.
- There are interactions between nutrients and food components in the gastrointestinal tract.
- There are interactions between nutrients and secreted substances in the gastrointestinal tract.
- Gut flora may contribute to certain nutrients, or may destroy them.
- There is also variation in absorptive capacity, feedback control of absorption by size of tissue load of nutrients.
- With respect to metabolism, there is variation in the distribution of nutrients across different tissues, including temporal effects involving the exchange of biochemicals across different body pools.
- There is variation in degradation of nutrients and in their excretory pathways.

Thus, although the use of biomarkers appears attractive, single measurements are often not adequate to provide accurate estimates of the excretion of any dietary component or nutrient of interest. In addition, standard methods for the use of biomarkers in dietary intake studies have yet to be widely accepted.

## Conclusion

This chapter presents a general overview of methods for studying dietary intake. These have been grouped according to the types of question that anthropologists

***Table 9.4.*** Recommendations for the design and analysis of diet studies (after the BGA Commission on Nutritional Epidemiology 1993)

| Study and analysis domain | Recommendations |
| --- | --- |
| Design of nutritional studies, including validation | Try to define the time period and the level of intake of the food or nutrient of interest, as a determinant of at risk. |
| | When designing a validation study, take into account the assessment of how good the method is at estimating the dietary intake of interest, and correction for misclassification of individuals according to their dietary intakes. |
| | Find an appropriate reference method for comparison, when estimating the amount of measurement error. |
| | A validation study should include the test method and a reference method which is essentially different from the test method, in the sense that it is reasonable to believe that the measurement errors are uncorrelated. |
| Validation of different study designs | In cohort studies, the validation subsample should be targeted at those strata which will yield the highest number of cases. |
| | For the comparability of cases and controls in case-control studies: in controls, the main study method must be applied first and any additional validation measurements subsequently. |
| Statistical investigation of the sampled data | Nutritionists/fieldworkers should work together. |
| | In the analysis of validation studies, use regression analysis, variance component analysis, analysis of covariance, and mean and covariance structure analysis. |
| | Sensitivity analysis should be carried out to check the dependence of assumptions concerning measurement errors. |

ask, and which relate to: food consumption, nutrient intake and nutritional status. These types of question reflect nested levels of analysis, in that while it is possible to measure food consumption without having to estimate either nutrient intake or nutritional status, it is not possible to estimate nutrient intake without measuring food consumption. Furthermore, it is not possible to estimate the adequacy of intake of specific nutrients without estimating nutrient intake. The choice of method or methods to be used should be made once the extent of appropriateness for the question or questions in hand, the accuracy, precision, complexity and cost (in time and money) of the techniques chosen, and the ease of subsequent interpretation of quantitative results have been considered. This is often not straightforward. While many components of dietary intake study are available 'off-the-shelf', the combination of questions posed, community or population under study, methods chosen and analysis undertaken will be unique in all cases, apart perhaps from multicentre epidemiological studies. It is therefore important to carry out this evaluation for every study in which dietary data collection is to be undertaken, and not to rely on 'off-the-shelf' solutions to dietary intake study.

## References

B.G.A. Commission on Nutritional Epidemiology (1993) Recommendations for the design and analysis of nutritional epidemiologic studies with measurement errors in the exposure variables, *European Journal of Clinical Nutrition*, 47(2), (supplement): S53–7.

Bates, C.J. and Thurnham, D.I. (1997) Biochemical markers of nutrient intake. In Margetts, B.M. and Nelson, M. (eds) *Concepts in Nutritional Epidemiology*, Oxford University Press, Oxford: 170–240.

Black, A.E. (1986) The use of recommended daily allowances to assess dietary adequacy. *Proceedings of the Nutrition Society*, 45, 369–81.

Black, A.E. (1999) *Dietary energy intake measurements: validations against energy expenditure*, PhD thesis, University of Ulster, Coleraine.

Black, A.E. (2001) Dietary assessment for sports dietetics, *Nutrition Bulletin*, 26: 29–42.

Cameron, M.E. and van Staveren, W.A. (1988) *Manual on Methodology for Food Consumption Studies*, Oxford University Press, Oxford.

Cole, T.J. (1997) Sampling, study size, and power. In Margetts, B.M. and Nelson, M. (eds.) Design Concepts in Nutritional Epidemiology, Oxford University Press, Oxford: 64–86.

Ferro-Luzzi, A. (1982) Meaning and constraints of energy intake studies in free-living populations. In Harrison, G.A. (ed.) *Energy and Effort*, Taylor and Francis, London:115–137.

Fox, R.H. (1953) *A study of the energy expenditure of Africans engaged in various activities, with special reference to some environmental and physiological factors which may influence the efficiency of their work*, PhD thesis, University of London, London.

Garine, I. de and Koppert, S. (1990) Social adaptation to season and uncertainty in food supply. In Harrison, G.A. and Waterlow, J.C. (eds) *Diet and Disease,* Cambridge University Press, Cambridge: 240–289.

Gibson, R.S. (1990) *Principles of Nutritional Assessment,* Oxford University Press, Oxford.

Johnston, F.E. (1987) *Nutritional Anthropology,* Alan R. Liss, New York.

Lissner, L., Stevens, J. and Levitsky, D.A.(1988) Variations in energy intake during the menstrual cycle: implications for food-intake research, *American Journal of Clinical Nutrition,* 48: 956–62.

Livingstone, M.B.E., Prentice, A.M., Strain, J.J., Coward, W.A., Black, A.E., Barker, M.E., McKenna, P.G. and Whitehead, R.G. (1990) Accuracy of weighed dietary records in studies of diet and health, *British Medical Journal,* 300: 708–12.

Margetts B.M. and Nelson, M. (1997) *Design Concepts in Nutritional Epidemiology,* Oxford University Press, Oxford.

Mertz, W., Tsui, J.C., Judd, J.T., Reiser, S., Hallfrisch, J., Morris, E.R., Steele, P.D. and Lashley, E. (1991) What are people really eating? The relation between energy intake derived from estimated diet records and intake determined to maintain body weight. *American Journal of Clinical Nutrition,* 54: 291–5.

Nelson, M., Black, A.E., Morris, J.A. and Cole, T.J. (1989) Between- and within-subject variation in nutrient intake from infancy to old age: estimating the number of days required to rank dietary intakes with desired precision, *American Journal of Clinical Nutrition,* 50: 155–67.

Pelto, G.H., Pelto, P.J. and Messer, E. (1989) *Research Methods in Nutritional Anthropology,* United Nations University Publications, Tokyo.

Tarasuk, V. and Beaton, G.H. (1991) Menstrual cycle patterns in energy and macronutrient intake, *American Journal of Clinical Nutrition,* 53: 442–7.

Ulijaszek, S.J. (1992a) Human energetics methods in biological anthropology, *Yearbook of Physical Anthropology,* 35: 215–42.

Ulijaszek, S.J. (1992b) Dietary and nutrient intakes of 25 Ningerum (New Guinea) adult males at two times of the year, *American Journal of Human Biology,* 4: 469–79.

Ulijaszek,S.J. and Strickland, S.S. (1993) *Nutritional Anthropology: prospects and perspectives,* Smith-Gordon, London.

West, C.E. and van Staveren, W. (1997) Food consumption, nutrient intake, and the use of food composition tables. In Margetts, B.M. and Nelson, M. (eds) *Design Concepts in Nutritional Epidemiology,* Oxford University Press, Oxford: 107–122.

Willett, W.C. (1990) *Nutritional Epidemiology,* Oxford University Press, Oxford.

Willett, W.C., Sampson, L., Stampfer, M.J., Rosner, B., Bain, C., Witschi, J., Hennekens, C.H. and Speizer, F.E. (1985) Reproducibility and validity of a semiquantitative food frequency questionnaire, *American Journal of Epidemiology,* 122: 51–65.

# 10. STUDYING FOOD INTAKE FREQUENCY
## A MACROSURVEY TECHNIQUE FOR ANTHROPOLOGISTS

*Jeya Henry* and *Helen Macbeth*

## Introduction

The quantification and assessment of dietary intake may seem to the uninitiated to be a simple matter of observation and measurement. However, no area of nutritional research has been so problematic as the measurement of food intake in free living populations. Today, eating habits not only vary between different nations and different cultures, but they have also dramatically changed over time. Simple dietary intake records cannot encompass all of the variables that have direct impact on consumption and its quantification (Cameron and van Staveren 1988). Nonetheless, significant progress has been made and methods for assessing dietary intake have been well researched in order to identify their varying practical uses, limitations and applications (see Burke 1947, Block *et al.* 1986, Ulijaszek this volume).

This chapter will make the distinction between the anthropologist's interest in population studies and the interest of the more physiological nutritionist who is frequently content with smaller numbers, but requires considerable detail in regards to quantity and nutrient quality. We shall first provide a very brief summary of the more precise methods used by nutritionists and others to provide detailed records of food intake from which quantification of nutrients and/or energy intake can be calculated. We shall then proceed to describe in detail one macrosurvey method for studying 7-day food intake frequency, which is highly appropriate for meeting some anthropological objectives. It has proved inexpensive and useful when the objective was simply to compare the food patterns of two groups of people. Here the aim was not nutritional

precision, but an initial quantitative overview of foods eaten. This may usefully accompany qualitative ethnographic and anthropological research and/or
epidemiological research, especially in the comparison of populations, for,
even with participant observation (see Hubert this volume), the researcher
cannot be in every kitchen and dining room of a study population all the time.
This 7-day food intake frequency study method can also be used as a pilot
study prior to more detailed nutritional research, as it will indicate foods and
drinks more frequently consumed. Furthermore, the method is low cost and
the data can be gathered by one fieldworker with limited time in the field.

## Summary of Food Intake Survey Methods used by Nutritionists and Dieticians

In this section we briefly introduce some of the traditional survey methods
used by those involved in nutritional research. The following are broadly
ranked in decreasing order of precision.

- *Duplicate analysis method*: All foods and drinks are weighed and
  measured, and duplicate weighed samples are taken at the same time
  for chemical analysis. The only errors that may occur in this method
  would be due to sampling or laboratory errors. This method would
  provide very detailed and complete information, but is clearly costly in
  terms of both researcher and respondent time.
- *Precise weighing method*: All ingredients for cooked food and all other
  foods and drinks are weighed. Cooked foods are weighed again before
  serving, and all plate waste and discarded food is also weighed and
  recorded. Nutrient intakes are calculated from food composition tables.
  Errors due to use of food composition tables occur where the item is not
  exactly comparable to that in the table. However, by weighing individual ingredients, errors due to differences in the recipe are avoided.
- *Weighed inventory method*: All food and drink is weighed before eating,
  and waste and discarded food also. Again food tables are used for calculation of nutrients. Some cooked foods may be analysed or simply have
  their water contents determined. In this method, possibilities of 'recipe
  error' must now be added to 'food table error'.
- *Diary methods*: The subjects keep a diary and a survey worker or enu-
  merator helps them to do so to a greater or lesser extent. To assist the
  non-specialist, foods are recorded in measures that are familiar in the
  household, such as in cups, tablespoons or teaspoons or in other common
  units, such as slices of bread, fistfuls of rice, chapattis, peeled bananas,
  eggs, etc. Alternatively, portion sizes may be judged by reference to
  photographs, plastic models of food helpings, geometric shapes or simply
  described, and then an attempt is made to derive food weights. The enu-
  merator then has the task of calibrating these measures with metric

measures to derive the weights of foods consumed. Errors introduced here are many. They include the reliability, memory, literacy of the subject, as well as their attitude to the survey and its need for precision. Furthermore, error can derive from the calibration of the household measures and units in calculating the food weights, as well as from 'recipe error' and 'food table error'.

- *Recall: specific period*: The subjects, or one of their relatives, are each questioned about food intake during a given period prior to the interview, usually the previous twenty-four hours. The record is again usually given in familiar household measures and units (see also González and Mataix this volume) and again an attempt is made to derive food weights. To the errors listed in the above methods, errors introduced here relate to the memory and cooperation of the recaller and any biases due to the day chosen, for example due to differences between days of the week.

- *Recall: habitual intake*: The subjects or one of their relatives are each asked to describe their usual eating pattern. Commonly this is phrased in terms of how many times per day, per week or per month, they eat one particular or several named food items. Again measurement is attempted in units familiar to the respondents. The data may be used to construct a 'dietary pattern'. However, this method more than all those above is liable to be overladen, consciously or unconsciously, with material that the speaker deems appropriate to report (see also Medina this volume).

The description of 'food intake frequency' can be applied to the last three of the methods summarised above where frequency is recorded and estimations of portion sizes are made by the respondent. However, outlined below is a food intake frequency method where no attempt is made to assess portion size, weight or nutrient quantity. There are many publications on methods for surveying food intake for nutritional, dietary and epidemiological research, (e.g. Bingham 1987, Thompson and Byers 1994, Willett 1994), and the reader is advised to study these to obtain more information on the methods in the above summary (see also Ulijaszek this volume).

## Objectives for Collecting Precisely Measured Food Intake Data

In general, food intake studies are used to estimate the respondent's usual food intake. As discussed by Ulijaszek (this volume) one objective of such detailed intake surveys is to quantify nutrients and the reader will find that his discussion covers some of the problems and sources of error associated with such research. As his chapter goes on to explain, the quantification of nutrient intake may well be for the purpose of measuring nutritional status, and he outlines further complexities in this analysis.

Another aspect in the study of nutritional status is the study of 'Energy Balance'. Energy balance is described by the simple equation:

***ENERGY BALANCE = ENERGY INTAKE – ENERGY EXPENDITURE***

Methods to estimate energy expenditure are described by Pasquet in the next chapter, but energy intake of course is derived largely from food. Energy is conventionally measured using either of two alternative units, kilocalories or kilojoules. In order to translate the amounts of food consumed into energy units, exact measurement and quantification of food intake are again needed. The precise food quantities are multiplied by energy equivalents of the various food items, and these energy equivalents can be found in food composition tables (e.g. Food Standards Agency 2002). For establishing energy intake, as for other nutrient intake, the most precise values are obtained from the 'duplicate analysis method', described above. However, in reality most nutritionists and anthropologists use a combination of methods, as appropriate to the circumstances where the data are to be gathered (e.g. Panter-Brick 1990). For example for literate populations recall over a specific period and diary methods are appropriate, but inappropriate in non-literate populations. Whilst it is impossible to obtain absolutely precise values at the individual level with these methods, the measures nevertheless can provide a useful insight into the energy intake of a population to be compared with the measures of their energy expenditure. Energy flow diagrams have been used to show how energy is consumed and expended in a small population (see, for example, Thomas 1976). Although it is hard to claim absolute kilocalorie precision for these energy flow diagrams, they have illuminated links and processes useful for the assessment of energy balance in a population.

All the methods for nutritional research referred to in this and the previous chapter are more fully explained in other published texts, and it is important to recognise that there is no single 'best' method for assessing dietary intake. Each method possesses certain advantages and one of the most important points to remember is that the objective of any study for which dietary information is desired must be clearly defined. The objective determines the appropriate method to be employed in collecting, processing and interpreting dietary data. It has been shown that this point has not always been appreciated by researchers.

## Food Intake Frequency Surveys

One significant reason for considering the objective carefully is that for some purposes a full survey of weighed and measured food intake may not be needed. Dietary surveys as described above are labour-intensive. In a survey where one observer is needed to weigh each subject's food, each observer can only work with a maximum of three subjects for the period surveyed. Even where the food is not weighed, but the respondent assesses the measures or units, the data, whether observed or recorded or acquired through interview, take considerably longer to collect than when the frequency of consumption of each food or drink item is simply recorded unmeasured. In the latter surveys the *frequency* of intake of each item becomes the relevant data, but not the provision of exact or estimated measurement of amount of nutrient or energy intake. Food frequencies may be recorded in diaries, by recall for a specific period or by recall for habitual intake. Points made above about problems arising in each of these methods should also be noted in relation to such methods of studying food intake frequency (Mullen and Krantzer 1984, Willett *et al.* 1985).

Since for anthropological studies the objective is usually to assess the intake of groups of people rather than of individuals, the time factor becomes highly significant. As the main cost items in any dietary survey will probably be the salaries, travel and subsistence of researchers and their assistants, their time is highly significant for research budgets. Food intake frequency methods, without estimates of portion sizes, take much less time and are therefore likely to be considerably cheaper. However, it is essential to recognise the limitations of only studying frequency for many nutritional research purposes, while their advantages for pilot studies and overviews of population differences in food consumption behaviour may be particularly relevant to certain objectives of anthropological research.

## One Low-budget, 7-day Food Intake Frequency Macrosurvey Method

The rest of this chapter is devoted to one 7-day food intake frequency method which can be used to study a population, yet it can be carried out by one researcher in the field for ten days. Although there have been requests before that this method be made available to others, it has not been previously published and we are, therefore, describing the method in great detail. We, of course, believe that it should not stand alone, but be supported by information from longer term participant observation, household interviews, supermarket surveys, local magazines, etc., but these depend to some extent on the objective of the research. The method is based on a wide distribution of a food intake frequency record sheet, which is simple to complete, but was less simple to design.

### Designing the 7-day Food Intake Frequency Record Sheet

The method discussed here was developed (Macbeth 1995) to compare the food intake of two populations as part of a larger study of those populations, but the study had to be achieved with limited time and funding. The two populations were in one Pyrenean valley but divided by an international border. Despite different nationalities, there were some claims of unity through Catalan ethnicity and through residency within one valley surrounded by mountains. The question was whether the food habits of the two national sectors of this same valley were indeed alike or different. The survey was in association with a longer term study of the populations in that valley. Reasonable sample sizes were more important than detailed information on quantity and quality of nutrients and energy. The study was scheduled to avoid special fast or feast days. Concurrently a short period of participant observation and of household surveys was carried out in each population.

It was decided that the information from each respondent should cover seven days, thereby including five weekdays and a week end. The method of a 7-day diary was rejected because of the considerable extra work in making the verbal information across such diaries uniform for numeric analysis, especially when, as in this valley, three languages were involved (Catalan, French and Spanish). However, the use of recall methods was also rejected. Recall can be a poor representation of reality even for the previous twenty-four hours, and could certainly not be trusted for seven days. Also with only one researcher, there would only be time for a limited number of recall interviews. Instead, a 7-day record sheet was designed.

This record sheet was designed with food and drink items listed down the left hand column, grouped in categories familiar to modern households in Europe. For example, *potatoes* were grouped with *vegetables*, rather than with *carbohydrates*, whereas the latter category included both *bread* and *pasta*. Because of the researcher's general interest in health variables, cooking oils and fats were included. It was also thought to be important that only one sheet of paper, printed on both sides, should be involved, and the print had to be clearly readable. So, choice and limitation of items to be either individually named or given group categories was a significant issue to resolve. Local advice on that choice was sought. Careful study of the use of the translated words was undertaken by interviewing local housewives in each language prior to distribution of the forms. It was also helpful that many of these housewives were bilingual and some trilingual. They were excellent informants on equivalent meanings.

In the first study for which this method was designed it was thought that time of day of consumption would be a useful variable, and seven *time-of-day* columns were spread across the page. However, it turned out that columns for *day of the week* were far more useful as these showed both whether the seven days were completed and any week day/weekend differences as well. It was decided that the seven days could commence on any day of the week, so long as this was recorded. Space was left down the right hand margin of the record sheet for any further coding by the researcher.

Figures 10.1a and 10.1b provide an example of the questionnaire in English. All that the respondent need do is place a single vertical mark every time a food or drink item is consumed along the row of that item and in the column for the day of the week. There is no attempt to gain information on size of portion. Subsequent data entry on to computer becomes simple as the sum of vertical marks in each square of the matrix. Computer readable forms can be envisaged but have not been tried; one reason that with current technology these are unlikely to be viable is because the forms are carried around for seven days by respondents of different age groups. They are folded and become pretty scruffy. In our research, the forms were simply copied on to sheets of paper. Four different colours of paper were used for colour-coding (see below).

## Population Sampling and Distribution

Decisions about how to sample a population and how to reach that sample must be taken. Where the research budget is as limited as was the case in this research, door-to-door interviewing and delivery of the forms to a large sample size was out of the question. Our attention turned to places where people attended. It was felt that distribution through doctors' surgeries and the one hospital might lead to biased samples and health-conscious reporting of the food intake. It was decided that distribution would be undertaken through the secondary schools, and in a European context we recommend this method for inexpensive but wide dissemination of material. The links with the population became the teenagers (aged eleven to fourteen) themselves. The drawback is that the age distribution of respondents is not random. However, by using the colour-coding of the record sheets as yellow for the teenager, pink for the mother of that teenager, blue for the father and orange for any local grandparent, a cross-section of ages was at least achieved. The complexity of modern household formations necessitates that children understand that the form for a missing parent or parents did not have to be filled in or should be filled in by the appropriate adults *in loco parentis*.

In the first study in the Pyrenean valley one large secondary school on the French side of the border and three schools on the Spanish side (because of an age break between Spanish schools) were chosen. In subsequent comparative studies – one study in the Mediterranean coastal region either side of Franco-Spanish border, another in Mallorca and one in Scotland – it has always been possible to find one State school for each population to cover the relevant ages. In each study an agreement was first sought from the school principals that they would be willing to allow the study. Then arrangements were made whereby Macbeth addressed each class of teenagers between the ages of eleven and fourteen giving a very general talk about why nutrition is important for health. The time allotted to Macbeth for each class was usually one school 'period', normally allotted either to biology or to home economics, and the talk had to be brief. The record sheets were laid out in piles of each colour somewhere convenient, e.g. on the front desk, as well as a sheet for a preferences game (green) and an instruction sheet (white) with a brief questionnaire about type of parental home, occupation, language, etc. on the back.

***Figure 10.1a***   Example of 7-day Food Intake Frequency Record form, page 1

**7-DAY FOOD INTAKE FREQUENCY RECORD**                          No._____

Name of pupil_____ age of pupil_____ sex of pupil_____

| FOOD ITEMS | Day 1 | Day 2 | Day 3 | Day 4 | Day 5 | Day 6 | Day 7 |
|---|---|---|---|---|---|---|---|
| White bread | | | | | | | |
| Wholemeal bread | | | | | | | |
| Buns, croissants, etc. | | | | | | | |
| Dry biscuits, crispbread, etc. | | | | | | | |
| Other alternative to bread | | | | | | | |
| Did you put butter on? | | | | | | | |
| Did you put margarine on? | | | | | | | |
| ....jam/honey/marmelade? | | | | | | | |
| ....peanut butter/nuttela? | | | | | | | |
| ....cheese? | | | | | | | |
| ....other? | | | | | | | |
| **Carbohydrates** | | | | | | | |
| Breakfast cereals | | | | | | | |
| Rice | | | | | | | |
| Pasta (spaghetti/macaroni,etc.) | | | | | | | |
| Other | | | | | | | |
| **Vegetables** | | | | | | | |
| Lettuce | | | | | | | |
| Greens (cabbage,etc.) | | | | | | | |
| Peas | | | | | | | |
| Green beans | | | | | | | |
| White & other dry beans | | | | | | | |
| Lentils, split peas | | | | | | | |
| Corn, maize | | | | | | | |
| Potatoes | | | | | | | |
| Carrots, other roots | | | | | | | |
| Onions, leeks, etc. | | | | | | | |
| Other vegetable (which?        ) | | | | | | | |
| Was garlic used in cooking? | | | | | | | |
| **Meats** | | | | | | | |
| Beef, veal | | | | | | | |
| Hamburger | | | | | | | |
| Lamb, mutton | | | | | | | |
| Pork | | | | | | | |
| Ham, bacon, etc. | | | | | | | |
| Sausages, hotdogs, etc. | | | | | | | |
| Salami, pork pies, etc. | | | | | | | |
| Game | | | | | | | |
| Chicken | | | | | | | |
| Turkey/other poultry | | | | | | | |
| Other meat | | | | | | | |
| **Fish** | | | | | | | |
| White fish | | | | | | | |
| Oily fish (eg.mackerel) | | | | | | | |
| Shell fish | | | | | | | |
| Other fish (which?        ) | | | | | | | |
| **Other 'proteins'** | | | | | | | |
| Eggs, egg dishes | | | | | | | |
| Cooked cheese dishes | | | | | | | |

*Figure 10.1b* Example of 7-day Food Intake Frequency Record form, page 2

| Continued | Day 1 | Day 2 | Day 3 | Day 4 | Day 5 | Day 6 | Day 7 |
|---|---|---|---|---|---|---|---|
| **Dairy (not liquid)** | | | | | | | |
| Uncooked cheese | | | | | | | |
| Yoghurt, etc. | | | | | | | |
| Other (not drinks) | | | | | | | |
| **Soups** | | | | | | | |
| Home made soup | | | | | | | |
| Tinned soup | | | | | | | |
| Packet soup | | | | | | | |
| **Fruits** | | | | | | | |
| Fresh fruit | | | | | | | |
| Bottled/tinned fruit | | | | | | | |
| Frozen fruit | | | | | | | |
| Dried fruit | | | | | | | |
| Other fruit | | | | | | | |
| **Sweets, puddings, etc.** | | | | | | | |
| Ice cream | | | | | | | |
| Custards, instant whips, etc. | | | | | | | |
| Cakes etc. | | | | | | | |
| Biscuits,shortbread,etc. | | | | | | | |
| Sweets,chocolates,etc. | | | | | | | |
| Other sweet item | | | | | | | |
| **Did you add sugar?** | | | | | | | |
| **Extras, Nibbles, etc.** | | | | | | | |
| Nuts | | | | | | | |
| Crisps, salty nibbles | | | | | | | |
| Olives | | | | | | | |
| **Drinks –Please remember to mark these –** | | | | | | | |
| Milk drinks (hot or cold) | | | | | | | |
| . Full cream | | | | | | | |
| . Semi-skimmed | | | | | | | |
| . Skimmed | | | | | | | |
| . Flavoured milk | | | | | | | |
| Coffee | | | | | | | |
| Tea | | | | | | | |
| Did you add milk? | | | | | | | |
| Did you add sugar? | | | | | | | |
| Herbal tea | | | | | | | |
| Fruit juice | | | | | | | |
| Fizzy drink | | | | | | | |
| Wine | | | | | | | |
| Beer or cider | | | | | | | |
| Spirits, liqueur, 'hard' liquor | | | | | | | |
| Other alcohol | | | | | | | |
| Water | | | | | | | |
| Other drink (which?        ) | | | | | | | |
| | | | | | | | |
| | | | | | | | |

**If you have eaten or drunk anything else that you found hard to categorise in the list above, please list it below.**

| | | | | | | | |
|---|---|---|---|---|---|---|---|
| | | | | | | | |

The teenagers simply picked up one sheet of each colour and returned to their desks.

For the school children, these classes were a break from normal school routine and a cheerful atmosphere tended to reign, punctuated at times by some amusement at the speaker's imperfect use of the relevant language! This atmosphere was used to encourage cooperation. Students were asked to write *their own names*, age and class on the top of *every* questionnaire sheet, not parental names. Then they were asked to take the yellow sheet and write '*Mine*' on it, to write '*Mother*' on the pink sheet and '*Father*' on the blue sheet. For the orange sheet, they were asked to find either a grandparent of either sex, or an elderly neighbour.

The green sheet for the 'preferences game' will not be discussed here (but see Macbeth and Mowatt this volume, where the preferences game is described). What is important here is that this game is played in class in order to teach the teenagers how to mark a record sheet in the relevant column with one small vertical mark and not with a tick or a cross. Understanding this becomes important for the task of completing the food intake frequency record sheets. A brief overview of this task was then given, and the students were asked to take the yellow form ('*Mine*'), and mark on it the current day of the week. Under the first column for *Day 1* they then had to mark up what they had con- sumed so far that day. Most found the food items on the form quite quickly and were asked to put one vertical mark in the column of *Day 1* for that item, whether it had been a small helping or large. They were reminded about drinks and asked to find on the form where drinks were listed. They were reminded to be honest about snacks, but we think that in fact snacks were often omitted.

With most teenagers being able to understand this much with very little trouble, they were asked if they thought they could explain how to fill in forms to those *in loco parentis*. They were asked to stress to their parents that it was a serious study and that their help would be valuable, but of course not com- pulsory. It was made clear that not only was cooperation voluntary but also that it in no way affected the child's marks at school. The students were asked to append a note if they had a sibling in the same study and if so only submit one set of parental forms. In this way, in the first study, Macbeth was able to distribute about 3,000 forms in three to four days of addressing school chil- dren. The students were asked to bring back all their forms to a named teacher in their school exactly eight days later. In the first study about two thirds of the forms were returned, but many were quite empty. About one third (1,000) appeared at first glance to be fully completed and of these approximately two thirds were deemed to be valid, i.e. approximately 650 valid 7-day food intake frequency records. Although this seems like a large proportion lost or invalid, nevertheless to collect 650 forms deemed valid for a 7-day continuous and rather tedious chore for the respondent, in such a short period of time, is highly cost-effective. In subsequent studies, in one school the valid response rate was far worse, but in all others it was considerably better. Much seems to depend on teacher support and the willingness for students to cooperate with that teacher. Researchers, therefore, should take care to liaise well with teachers. Apart from forms either not returned or returned blank, the main reason for invalidity was that the respondent gave up after four or five days. This may make one return to the discussion above about the appropriate number of days for a useful intake frequency study, but European populations today do tend to have 7-day patterns in their food consumption behaviour and we still recommend 7-day studies.

## Getting Data Ready for Analysis

The data are received in matrix format on the respondent forms. Each school-child is given an individual code number, indicating the population, the school, the class and the individual. A suffix digit is added to distinguish the family roles of the student, the mother, the father and the elderly relative or neighbour. The identification of each case uses this composite code number, but no names are entered on to computer or become available to third parties. The variables of the child's age and sex are also coded and whether there is a sibling, especially a twin. Each variable column in the matrix is given a code-name, e.g. *Carrots1, Carrots2, Carrots3,* etc. for each day of the seven days, and the data (the sum of the vertical marks) in each square can be entered on computer using Excel, SPSS or whatever data entry program the researcher prefers.

There are various calculations now possible, but we shall describe those for total 7-day intake frequency. For each food or drink item a total frequency of consumption of that item during the seven days can be calculated. Further variables can be created; for example, food items can be grouped in categories, e.g. *red meat* or *total meat.* Consumption either of individual items or of these grouped categories can then be compared between population samples, or the categories themselves can be compared, for example frequency of consumption of *red meat* can be compared to that of *poultry.* Furthermore, any category can be made into a proportion, providing yet another variable, so that *red meat* as a proportion of *total meat* can be compared to the *poultry* proportion, etc. Proportions may be very useful variables for population comparisons where total intake frequencies diverge. The family role digits can also be used as variables, from which some rough indications of generational differences and/or family commensality can be gained.

## Statistical Analysis

It may be tempting simply to compare the means of intake frequencies of each food variable, but the distributions of the variables are far from Gaussian. There will be many individuals with a frequency of zero for many food items, with the exception probably of bread. Macbeth and assistants decided to use two other methods of statistical analysis.

Each population was divided between those who consumed the item one or more times and those who did not consume it even once. Simple chi-square analysis was then used for a matrix of percentages of 'who ate' and percentages of 'who did not even eat the item once', by any two populations to be compared. This is a simple analysis for revealing population differences. However, in order not to lose the information on frequency differences among those who did consume an item, Mann Whitney rank order analysis was also chosen. For both of these methods of analysis highly significant differences between the populations being studied were demonstrated (see, for example, Macbeth 1995). Further statistical methods and graphic displays can also be explored, but do not belong in this chapter. [For a useful introductory book for those who have not studied any statistics we recommend Rees (2001)]

## Some Results

What was particularly interesting in regard to the Catalan studies, in which this food intake frequency method was first used, was that prior oral information from locals might have lead the researcher to believe that there were essentially no food intake differences in the Pyrenean valley either side of the border. Yet, the quantified data showed many big differences at a high level of statistical significance. This supports Medina's view (this volume) about biases in oral information. Another conclusion from such simple quantitative food intake frequency data in the Pyrenees, on the Mediterranean coast and on the Island of Mallorca, was a clear demonstration of divergence in their diet in the 1990s from the Anglo-American concept of a 'Mediterranean Diet' (Macbeth 1998). Finally, the method was used to demonstrate that, for example, French/Spanish differences exceeded mountain/coastal differences in the four 'populations' studied in Catalonia.

These few reported results are only included to indicate the kind of conclusions for which these low-cost data are adequate, but this method should never be used to replace more costly and more detailed nutritional information where this is needed and can be afforded. At best the method would provide a useful pilot study for those interested in nutritional status or energy balance, while it may be extremely useful for some of the broader objectives of anthropological research.

## Conclusion

The reader has been briefly introduced to a summary of methods used by nutritionists for studying food intake, the details of all of which can be pursued in other published sources. The need to assess both qualitative and quantitative aspects of dietary intake has been repeatedly emphasised by nutritionists and health professionals, as well as by the anthropologists. In this chapter, however, emphasis has been given to detailed instructions for one, so far unpublished, method that many anthropologists might find useful to use for a low-cost macrosurvey. In this method nutrient and energy quantities remain unknown, but the results can identify trends, which may be of interest to cultural as well as biological anthropologists, epidemiologists, nutritionists and food scientists. Research objectives exist where it may be better to sacrifice in this way precision for a broader-based study within a limited budget. Once a population trend or pattern has been shown from such a study, it can be used to direct further investigation using different disciplinary methods for different purposes.

For some the method explained in detail in this chapter might be used for an inexpensive pilot study to justify an application for finance for a larger, more detailed nutritional study. For others it will be used in conjunction with participant observation, interviewing, household questionnaires and surveys of kitchens, larders, markets and supermarkets, in a review of food habits of one or more societies. An anthropologist pursuing a holistic approach may well find it useful to include this particular food intake frequency method within their research, in association with other methods and perspectives. The use of more than one method for a fuller illumination of a research question is stressed in several chapters in this book.

## Acknowledgements

The authors wish to thank Jacques and Hélène Vergé, Enric and Teresa Subirats, and the directors, staff and students at the secondary schools in Bourg Madame, Puigcerdà, Llansà, Port Bou, Port Vendres, Andraitx and Banchory, as well as all who completed the 7-day records. ESRC grant no. R-000-232816 is acknowledged and Macbeth is very grateful for the assistance of Alex Green and Aleks Collingwood Bakeo for work in connection with designing the 7-day records. Helen Lightowler is thanked for reading the final draft.

## References

Bingham, S.A. (1987) The dietary assessment of individuals; methods, accuracy, new techniques and recommendations, *Nutrition Abstracts and Reviews*, 57(10): 705–42.

Block, G., Hartman, A.M., Dresser, C.M., Gannon, J. and Gardner, L. (1986) A data-based approach to diet questionnaire design and testing, *American Journal of Epidemiology*, 124: 453–469.

Burke, B.S. (1947) The diet history as a tool in research, *Journal of the American Dietetic Association*, 23: 1041–1046.

Cameron, M.E. and van Staveren, W.A. (1988) *Manual on Methodology for Food Consumption Studies*, Oxford University Press, Oxford.

Food Standards Agency (2002) *McCance and Widdowson's The Composition of Foods*, (sixth summary edition), Royal Society of Chemistry, Cambridge.

Macbeth, H.M. (1995), The Cerdanya, a valley divided: biosocial anthropology in a
    research project. In A.J.Boyce and V.Reynolds (eds) *Human Populations: diversity
    and adaptation*, Oxford University Press, Oxford: 231–251.
Macbeth, H.M. (1998), Concepts of 'The Mediterranean Diet' in U.K. and Australia
    compared to food intake studies on the Catalan coast of the Mediterranean, *Rivista
    di Antropologia*, 76 (Supplement): 307–13.
Mullen, B.J. and Krantzer, N.J. (1984) Validity of a food frequency questionnaire for
    the determination of individual food intake, *American Journal of Clinical Nutrition*,
    39: 136–143.
Panter-Brick, C. (1990) Field studies of energy balance. In Chapman, M. and
    Macbeth, H. *Food for Humanity*, Centre for the Sciences of Food and Nutrition,
    Oxford.
Rees, D. (2001) *Essential Statistics* (4th Edition), Chapman and Hall/CRC, New York.
Thomas, R.B. (1976) Energy flow at high altitude. In Baker, P.T. and Little, M.A.
    (eds) *Man in the Andes: A multidisciplinary study of high altitude Quechua*,
    Dowden, Hutchinson and Ross, Stroudsburg: 379–404.
Thompson, F.E. and Byers, T. (1994) Dietary assessment resource manual, *Journal of
    Nutrition*, 124(11) (supplement): 2245S–2317S.
Willett, W. (1994) Future directions in the development of food-frequency
    questionnaires, *American Journal of Clinical Nutrition*, 59 (supplement): 171s–174s.
Willett, W.C., Sampson, L., Stampfer, M.J., Rosner, B., Bain, C., Witschi, J.,
    Hennekens, C.H. and Speizer, F.E. (1985) Reproducibility and validity of a
    semiquantitative food frequency questionnaire, *American Journal of Epidemiology*,
    122: 51–65.

# 11. THE CONCEPT OF ENERGY BALANCE AND THE QUANTIFICATION OF TIME ALLOCATION AND ENERGY EXPENDITURE

*Patrick Pasquet*

## Introduction

An important concern for nutritionists and nutritional anthropologists is the balance between intake and expenditure of energy. This is referred to as *energy balance*. The relevance of this to food anthropologists is that energy intake is gained largely through food, and to those interested in nutritional status it is whether intake exceeds the expenditure or *vice versa*. In developed countries people are encouraged to understand that through control of intake and/or exercise they can modify that balance to gain or lose weight. However, anthropologists tend to be more interested in groups, 'populations' or 'societies' and the study of energy intake and expenditure through populations has been developed, and is referred to as *energy flow* studies. A pioneering and important example of such studies is the work by Thomas (e.g. 1976) and a useful proceedings volume on energy balance in humans was edited by Harrison (1982). There is reference to energy balance and energy intake through food in the previous chapter (Henry and Macbeth this volume). This chapter is primarily about the measurement of energy expenditure.

## The Measurement of Energy Expenditure

For several decades anthropologists have been increasingly concerned with how to measure time use, activity patterns and energy output at the individual, household and population levels. These data are essential elements for revealing the adaptive responses and strategies – biological, behavioural or cultural –

which humans use to cope with different situations of nutritional constraints (Blaxter and Waterlow 1985).

Quantifying time allocation and energy balance is used for resolving numerous and varied questions, such as information on the physiological and metabolic adaptations to the variations of energy availability (e.g. Ferro-Luzzi *et al.* 1990), and for activity-related behavioural responses to nutritional constraints (Gorsky and Calloway 1983). In children, the research can be about the study of relationships between activity level, growth, motor and cognitive development (Schürch and Scrimshaw 1990). It can also concern the study of work, effort and productivity in relation to nutritional status (Spurr 1983) and reproductive function (Rosetta 1993).

At the household/population level, activity-energy data can be used for understanding the relationship between social organisation, labour, income and nutritional outcome of all members within a community (Gross 1984). In an ecological perspective cross-cultural comparisons of the energy efficiency of subsistence strategies (e.g. Ulijaszek and Poraituk 1993) aid understanding of the dynamics of energy flows in particular environments (Bekerman 1993). They can also be used to test models and theories in the study of human cultural evolution (Hill 1982).

The assessment of activity and energy expenditure is also of practical value since it provides essential data for the debate on defining optimal food and nutritional needs, including energy needs (F.A.O./W.H.O./U.N.U. 1985). An important use of these data is in the field of medical anthropology, for instance in relation to the aetiology of nutrition related health disorders, such as obesity in affluent and transitional societies (Pearson 1990). Finally, time and energy data provide elements for testing the capacity of a given society to develop, as well as for assessing the impact of socio-economic development policies (Pasquet 1998) and malnutrition prevention programmes (Going *et al.* 1999).

This chapter describes the various field methods used for assessing time allocation and energy expenditure as used by anthropologists, human ecologists and others. Particular attention will be given to the relevance of each method in different research situations.

## Activity Patterns and Time Budgets

The activity of an individual can be indirectly quantified by the study of their time budget. Three categories of methods are in use according to whether one calls upon memory (retrospective questionnaires), self-assessment (diaries), or direct observation (continuous observation or random spot checks). Another, more indirect approach to studying activity involves methods using measurements of physiological or mechanical parameters (e.g. heart rate monitoring and motion sensors).

## Retrospective Questionnaires

Questionnaires are extensively used in nutritional epidemiology (Washburn and Montoye 1986) to provide information on the activity patterns of large groups. Methods using recall refer to activity of the previous days, week, season, year or any particular period of time (Boisvert *et al.* 1988). The questionnaire can be completed either by the subject or by an interviewer. The activities should be pre-coded into a reduced number of items. The duration may vary with the objective of the study, but should never exceed an hour. Reproducibility of questionnaires is useful but depends on the types of activity (Booth *et al.* 1996). Despite relatively weak accuracy, such questionnaires, used in an appropriate way, can make it possible to discriminate between groups and populations according to their patterns and levels of activity (Roeykens *et al.* 1998).

## Activity Diaries

In this method the subjects report on their activities in diaries over particular periods of time (Durnin and Passmore 1967). The interval between the reports is variable (every minute, five minutes, half hour, one hour, etc.) and is the result of a compromise between the precision of the information sought and the subject's availability and lassitude. Most of the time, the type of activity is pre-coded in order to simplify the report. Sometimes the activity level is recorded with the help of a scale of perceived exertion (Varghese *et al.* 1994). However, the diary technique requires significant cooperation from the surveyed person and is less appropriate for some populations. Moreover the activity report can interfere with the habitual activity and thus alter the representativeness of the data.

## Direct Observation

Activity patterns and level can be computed either from *continuous observation* (*time and motion studies* and *video recording*) or from *random observations* (*spots checks*).

*Time and motion*: in time and motion studies the activities of a focal individual (or a focal group of cooperating individuals) is continuously observed and recorded. This method has been extensively applied in the rural areas of developing countries, especially when the sense of time in the study population is not compatible with recall of this type of information (Norgan *et al.* 1974). Research assistants (local, where possible) record starting and stopping times for all activities during the waking day or during a particular window of time (serial observation). An alternative is minute by minute recording for a finite period of time. Two observers are necessary for this. The periods of observation can be from two to seven days according to the variability of the activities. For precision, the activity should be reported clearly; the use of codes facilitates recording but causes an additional workload for local assistants who are often little familiarised with this type of procedure. Additional information can be useful, such as posture of the focal subject(s), their walking pace, the load carried, and the local geography (e.g. the nature of the ground, the steepness of the incline in mountain areas, etc.). In traditional subsistence populations particular attention must be paid to the duration and paces involved in displacements. Displacements represented up to 25 percent of the energy budget in the forest population we studied in South Cameroon (Pasquet and Koppert 1993). These can be accurately quantified with the help of a portable Global Positioning System (GPS) receiver worn by the subject.

Time and motion studies undoubtedly allow the most exhaustive description of the activity of an individual over long periods. The technique is generally well accepted by those studied if the duration of observation is reasonable. It is nevertheless an expensive method in terms of staff and time, which either limits the study sample to a few individuals (defined by age, sex, productive or social categories) or requires a large budget. Another problem is that we cannot exclude the possibility that the presence of an observer can to some extent alter the habitual activity pattern of the person followed. However, a long-term stay in the field should make it possible to remove this uncertainty.

*Video Recordings*: audio-visual techniques – in particular video recordings – constitute a useful method for fine continuous observations of activities and behavioural interactions. They are particularly suitable for the observation of young children and analysis of their interactions with their environments. The technique is generally well accepted after a short period of adaptation. Moreover the low price of amateur video hardware now makes it relatively accessible. However, the examination of hours of filmed information afterwards is extremely tedious and requires technical skills and equipment.

*Random Spot Checks*: the so-called *random spot checking* method, developed by Johnson (1975), is an interesting alternative to continuous observation. Inexpensive and hardly invasive, this method has been adopted by ethnographers and geographers. It is particularly suited for studies undertaken at the level of a whole community. The method consists of noting the behaviours of individuals at particular instances using random sampling techniques. Typically, units (cooperating groups or households) are randomly chosen from a list of such units: they are then observed on a particular day and at a particular time of the day, also chosen at random. The observer arrives unexpectedly at the observation spot, where most of the unit members are expected to be observable, and writes down the activities carried out by those present. If all individuals in the observation unit are not observable within a given period of time (generally one hour), those present are interviewed about where the absent ones are and what their activities are likely to be at the observation time. Over a long period (a month, a season, a year), these data provide the researcher with a reliable sample of the activity patterns of all subjects. A sample of 600 to 700 observations is sufficient to establish a clear activity profile of a category of individuals within a community (Bernard and Killworth 1993). Quantification of daily energy expenditure, adjusting spot data to continuous observation of selected individuals provides a method that is efficient in terms of effort.

## Energy Expenditure

Only after having studied the activities, can the energy expenditure resulting from these activities be computed. Several approaches satisfy the requirements of field studies: the factorial method, heart rate monitoring, motion sensors, the doubly labelled water method and intake recording.

In the first place, account must be taken of the basal metabolism, the minimal energy expenditure for the maintenance of vital functions, growth, pregnancy and lactation, which is the largest component of total daily energy expenditure; it accounts for 50 to 70 percent of the value. The measurement of the basal metabolic rate (BMR), therefore, requires detailed attention. BMR is usually measured using *indirect calorimetry* to calculate oxygen consumption, but in practice it is customary to predict BMR using various equations (see below).

## Factorial Method

The factorial method has been extensively used in population-based energy expenditure studies (Durnin and Brockway 1959). It consists of integrating, over time, the caloric cost of the component activities, the duration of which will have been determined by direct observation, diaries or questionnaires. Information on the energy costs comes from measurements actually carried out in the field and/or from predicted values from the literature. Total daily energy expenditure (TDEE) is then computed by integrating the whole unit's activity energy costs over periods both of waking and of sleeping. It is agreed that one can consider the expenditure of energy during sleep as starting from the basal expenditure, the BMR. The factorial method, then, is the sum of other measurements, examples of which follow.

## Measurement of Activity Energy Cost

In practice, measurements relate to the most representative activities in the study group: single or standardised activities like resting, walking, load carrying, plus complex activities relevant to that society. It is advisable to take measurements several times on as many individuals as possible.

*Indirect Calorimetry* measures energy expenditure (Atwater and Benedict 1903) as the rate at which heat is produced by the body, i.e. the rate of respiratory gases exchange (i.e. oxygen uptake and/or production of carbon dioxide).

*The Douglas Bag Method* (Douglas 1911) is widely used in field studies. The Douglas bag collects and measures air exhaled. The measurement sessions last from five to fifteen minutes according to the type of activity. The gases are collected in bags of a capacity of 100 to 150 litres. Gases are then analysed in portable measuring equipment. For details of the calculation of the energy expenditure see McLean and Tobin (1987). During measurement, however, the embarrassment of carrying a cumbersome bag filled with air can deteriorate the representativeness of measurement, in particular for activites at high altitude.

*Other Portable Equipment* has been developed to replace Douglas bags, for example the *Kofranyi-Michaelis Respirometer* (Kofranyi and Michaelis 1940), which consists of a gas meter coupled to a system of sampling of the air expired for remote analysis of gases. Light (3kg) and robust, this simple mechanical instrument is appropriate for use in field settings but allows only measurements of relatively short duration. However it is no longer commercially available.

*Other Portable Lightweight Systems*, capable of measuring energy expenditure continuously for long periods, have been developed more recently, the *Oxylog* (P. K. Morgan Ltd, Rainham England), the *Cosmed K4b$^2$ system* (Cosmed, Pavona di Albano, Italy) and *the Total Energy Expenditure Measurement system* (TEEM 100, Aerosport, Ann Arbor, USA). All three systems integrate in the same instrument a gas meter and a gas analyser allowing the calculation of oxygen uptake. They are, moreover, equipped with a device for the storage of the data. Validity studies (Harrison *et al.* 1982, Segal *et al.* 1994, Hausswirth *et al.* 1997) have suggested that these instruments are sufficiently precise and faithful for the measurement of activity energy expenditure in laboratory conditions, but only the Oxylog has been extensively tested in various field conditions. However, the price of these instruments limits their use for large samples of individuals.

## Predictions and Use of Tables in the Literature

Activity energy cost can be estimated using either the formulas of prediction or data published in the literature. BMR can be predicted starting from the measurement of body weight using age/sex and population specific equations (e.g. Schofield 1985, Henry and Rees 1991). The metabolic cost of the other activities can be estimated using published tables (e.g. James and Schofield 1990, Ainsworth *et al.* 1993). Validity studies have shown that the factorial method allows accurate and reliable estimates of energy expenditure of groups of individuals (Warwick *et al.* 1988). Since the major potential source of bias of the method is in the value of the energy cost assigned to the various activities (Spurr *et al.* 1997) and in the capacity of the investigator to judge activity levels, it is advisable to measure actual energy expenditure whenever possible.

## Heart Rate Monitoring

This method uses the close linear relationship which binds the heart rate (HR) to the oxygen uptake during physical activity to predict energy expenditure (Booyens and Hervey 1960). Spurr *et al.* (1988) proposed the *Flex heart rate*. The method uses continuous minute-by-minute HR records (instead of average HR). The data are partitioned into two sets depending on whether HR is below or above a value named the *Flex point*, below which HR is no longer correlated to energy expenditure. This is presumed to establish the subject's individual heart rate *versus* oxygen uptake relationship. Measurements of resting expenditure and HR, including in various postures and at different times of the day, are performed. TDEE is estimated starting from the sum of the several components. Recently, reliable, lightweight and inexpensive devices for measuring HR have been introduced, which allow several days of continuous measurement, the storage and the direct restitution of the data on a computer after processing (e.g. S610 Polar heart rate monitor, Polar Electro, Kempele, Finland).

The HR method is socially acceptable and yields valuable data on activity patterns and level, and accurate estimates of mean group total energy expenditure for all sex-age categories (Livingstone *et al.* 1990). Despite resorting to indirect calorimetry, the necessity for individual calibration of the subjects and some other technical difficulties, the HR method has benefits which mean that it is increasingly used as a reference method not only in anthropological but also in medium-sized epidemiological studies (Wareham *et al.* 1997).

## Motion Sensors

Motion sensors are devices intended to quantify directly motor activity using biomechanical parameters, for example through movement counters and accelerometers. The pedometer is an example of a movement counter. Accelerometers (e.g. CSA accelerometer, Manufacturing Technology Inc., Fort Walton Beach, FL, USA) measure the accelerations and decelerations of the body and are thus supposed to provide a better account of differences in physical activity than movement counters (Westerterp 1999). The validity of accelerometers to predict habitual energy expenditure remains unclear (Hendelman *et al.* 2000). However the combined use of accelerometer and heart rate monitoring offers promise for the assessment of free-living physical activity and energy expenditure (Rennie *et al.* 2000).

## The Doubly-labelled Water Method

Developed in the 1950s, this method was first used in animals and validated for humans in the early 1980s (Schoeller and van Santen 1982). The technique consists of measuring the turnover of two isotopes: deuterium ($^2H$) and oxygen

18 ($^{18}$O) over a given period of time in order to estimate the quantity of carbon dioxide produced and thus the energy expended during this period of time. In practice doses of water marked by the two isotopes are orally administrated. Samples of urine are gathered every day during the whole measurement period (generally from one to two weeks) and finally the isotopic abundance is analysed in a mass spectrometer (for more details on the technique, see Prentice 1990).

## The Intake-balance Method

This method was for a long time the reference method for assessing daily energy expenditure (DEE) of free-living subjects. The approach combines the measurements of daily energy intake (DEI) and of variation in body energy stores ($\Delta$ES) according to the formula:

$$DEE = DEI \pm | \Delta ES |.$$

DEI is obtained from nutrient intake and $\Delta$ES is deduced from the variations of body composition by allotting a caloric equivalent per gram of fat and/or of lean body mass stored or mobilised. In a cross-disciplinary book such as this, details on such a method are of necessity greatly abbreviated and researchers are strongly advised to seek further information on methods for measuring energy intake and body composition from sources such as Jebb and Elia (1993) and Ulijaszek (1995). In the field, $\Delta$ESs can be approximated from the variation of body weight alone, which is considered to be a very reliable measurement. The caloric equivalent cost of the variations of body weight is a function of the subject's biological category (growing child, adult, pregnant or lactating woman, etc.) (FAO/WHO/UNU 1985).

One month appears to be the minimal duration of measurements necessary to establish a realistic assessment of energy balance. The precision of the intake-balance method depends on many factors (food recording method, consumption patterns in the target population, etc.), but one can consider 15 percent to be the mean error on the total daily energy expenditure of a group of twenty to fifty individuals (Ulijaszek 1992). This is an error higher than that of many other methods. Consequently the intake-balance method does not appear to be the most appropriate method to estimate energy output in anthropological studies. Furthermore, one must always be aware of the possibility of circular reasoning, when using energy intake and physiological variables to measure energy expenditure.

## Conclusion

Field research is always a compromise between the requirements of scientific rigour and what is realisable (taking into account budgetary constraints, time

***Table 11.1*** Ranking of methods for assessment of energy expenditure in field settings

| Method | Accuracy | Cost | Acceptance | Technical feasibility |
|---|---|---|---|---|
| factorial method | | | | |
| – tables and predictions | + | ++ | +++ | +++ |
| – calorimetry | ++ | + | ++ | ++ |
| heart rate recording | ++ | ++ | +++ | ++ |
| movement sensors | +(+) | +++ | +++ | +++ |
| heart rate + movement sensor | +++(+) | ++ | +++ | ++ |
| doubly-labelled water | ++++ | – | ++++ | + |
| Intake- balance | + | ++ | ++ | ++ |

++++ excellent, +++ very good, ++ good, + acceptable, – bad

allowed for the study and local human and physical contexts). There is no 'ideal method' for assessing activity budgets and energy expenditure ; the simplest techniques tend to be the least accurate and *vice versa*. Table 11.1 shows the ranking of methods used to assess energy expenditure in field settings, in terms of validity, applicability and cost.

Whatever the methods, they must be adapted to the objective of the study and to the characteristics of the target population. In any case, time use and energy studies should be preceded by the gathering of general information on the population, for example, the demographic structure, the household and social organisation, any seasonality in food procurement and production patterns, the educational level and the sense of time. It must be kept in mind that a long stay in the field will always stimulate better collaboration and willingness from the community members. As mentioned by Garine (this volume), collaboration with an ethnographer already familiar with the people and their society can be very beneficial.

# References

Ainsworth, B.E., Haskell, W.L., Leon, H.S., Jacobs Jr., D.R, Montoye, H.J., Sallis, J.F. and Paffenberger Jr., R.S. (1993) Compendium of physical activities: classification of energy costs of human physical activities, *Medicine and Science in Sports and Exercise*, 25: 71–80.

Atwater, W.O. and Benedict, F.G. (1903) *Experiments on the metabolism of matter and energy in the human body*, Office of Experimental Stations, Bulletin n°136, United States Department of Agriculture, Washington DC.

Bekerman, S. (1993) Major patterns in indigenous amazonian subsistence. In Hladik, C.M., Hladik, A., Linares, O.F., Pagézy, H., Semple, A. and Hadley, M. (eds).

*Tropical Forests, People and Food: Biocultural Interactions and Applications to Development*, Man and the Biosphere series, 13, Unesco, Paris: 411–424.

Bernard, R.H. and Killworth, P.D. (1993) Sampling in time allocation research, *Ethnology*, 27: 155–179.

Blaxter,K and Waterlow J.C., (1985) *Nutritional adaptation in man*, John Libbey, London.

Boisvert, P., Washburn, R.A., Montoye, H.J. and Leger, L. (1988) Mesure et évaluation de l'activité physique par questionnaire. Questionnaires utilisés dans la littérature anglo-saxonne, *Science & Sports*, 3: 245–262.

Booth, M.L., Owen, N., Bauman, A.E. and Gore, C.J. (1996) Retest reliability of recall measures of leisure-time physical activity in Australian adults, *International Journal of Epidemiology*, 25: 153–159.

Booyens, J. and Hervey, G.R. (1960) The pulse rate as a means of measuring metabolic rate in man, *Canadian Journal of Biochemical Physiology*, 38: 1301–1309.

Douglas, C.G. (1911) A method for determining the total respiratory exchange in man, *Journal of Physiology*, 42: xvii–xviii.

Durnin, J.V.G.A. and Brockway, J.M. (1959) Determination of the total daily energy expenditure in man by indirect calorimetry: assessment of the accuracy of a modern technique, *British Journal of Nutrition*, 13: 41–53.

Durnin, J.V.G.A. and Passmore, R. (1967) *Energy, work and leisure*, Heinemann Educational Books, London.

F.A.O./W.H.O./U.N.U. (1985) *Energy and protein requirements*, Technical report no 724; WHO, Geneva.

Ferro-Luzzi, A., Scaccini, C., Taffese, S., Aberra, B. and Demeke, T. (1990) Seasonal energy deficiency in Ethiopian rural women, *European Journal of Clinical Nutrition*, 44 (Suppl. 1): 7–18.

Going, S.B., Levine, S., Harell, J., Stewart, D., Kushi, L., Cornell, C.E., Hunsberger, S., Corbin C. and Sallis J. (1999) Physical activity assessment in American Indian schoolchildren in the Pathways study, *American Journal of Clinical Nutrition*, 69: 788S–795S.

Gorsky, R.D. and Calloway, D.H. (1983) Activity pattern change with decrease in energy intake, *Human Biology*, 55: 577–586.

Gross, D.R. (1984) Time allocation: a tool for the study of cultural behavior, *Annual Reviews of Anthropology*, 13: 519–558.

Harrison, G.A., (1982) (ed.) *Energy and Effort*, Taylor and Francis, London.

Harrison, M.H., Brown, G.A. and Belyavin, A.J. (1982) The 'Oxylog': an evaluation. *Ergonomics*, 25: 809–820.

Haußwirth, C., Bigard, A.X. and Le Chevalier, J.M. (1997) The Cosmed K4 telemetry system as an accurate device for oxygen uptake measurements during exercise, *International Journal of Sports Medicine*, 18: 449–453.

Hendelman, D., Miller, K., Bagget, C., Debold, E., Freedson, P. and Montoye, H.J. (2000) Validity of accelerometry for the assessment of moderate activity in the field, *Medicine and Science in Sports and Exercise*, 32, (supplement): S442–S449.

Henry, C.J.K. and Rees, D.G. (1991) New predictive equations for the estimation of basal metabolic rate in tropical peoples, *European Journal of Clinical Nutrition*, 45: 177–185.

Hill, K. (1982) Hunting and human evolution. *Journal of Human Evolution*, 11: 521–44.

Jebb, S.A. and Elia, M. (1993) Techniques for the measurement of body composition: a practical guide, *International Journal of Obesity*, 17: 611–621.

Johnson, A. (1975) Time allocation in a Machiguenga Community, *Ethnology*, 14: 301–310.

Kofranyi, E and Michaelis, H.F. (1940) Ein tragbarer apparat zur bestimmung des gasstoffwechsels, *Arbeitsphysiologie*, 11: 148–150.

Livingstone, M.B.E., Prentice, A.M., Coward, W.A., Ceesay, S.M., Strain, J.J., McKenna, P.G., Nevin, G.B., Barker, M.E. and Hichey, R.J. (1990) Simultaneous measurement of free-living energy expenditure by the doubly labeled water method and heart rate monitoring, *American Journal of Clinical Nutrition*, 52: 59–65.

McLean, J.A and Tobin, G. (1987) *Animal and Human Calorimetry*, Cambridge University Press, Cambridge.

Norgan, N.G., Ferro-Luzzi, A. and Durnin, J.V.G.A. (1974) The energy and nutrient intake and the energy expenditure of 204 New Guinean adults, *Philosophical transactions of the Royal Society of London*, B268: 309–348.

Pasquet, P. (1998) Ethnoecology: results from studies on time allocation and daily activities. *APFT- News*, 5: 3–4.

Pasquet, P. and Koppert, G.J.A. (1993) Activity patterns and energy expenditure in cameroonian tropical forest populations. In Hladik, C.M., Hladik A., Linares O.F., Pagézy H., Semple A. and Hadley M. (eds) *Tropical Forests, People and Food: Biocultural Interactions and Applications to Development*, Man and the Biosphere series, Unesco, volume 13, Paris: 311–320.

Pearson, J. (1990) Estimation of energy expenditure in Western Samoa, American Samoa and Honolulu by recall interviews and direct observation, *American Journal of Human Biology*, 2: 313–326.

Prentice, A.M. (1990) *The Doubly-Labelled Water Method for Measuring Energy Expenditure. Technical Recommandations for use in Humans*, IDECG/IAEA, NAHRES-4, Vienna.

Rennie, K., Rowsell, T., Jebb, S.A., Holburn, D. and Wareham, N.J. (2000) A combined heart rate and movement sensor: proof of concept and preliminary testing study. *European Journal of Clinical Nutrition*, 54: 409–414.

Roeykens, J., Rogers, R., Meeusen, R., Magnus, L., Borms, J. and de Meirleir, K. (1998) Validity and reliability in a Flemish population of the WHO-MONICA optional study of physical activity questionnaire, *Medicine and Science in Sports and Exercise*, 30: 1071–1075.

Rosetta, L. (1993) Female reproductive dysfunction and intense physical training, *Oxford Reviews of Reproductive Biology*, 15: 113–141.

Schoeller, D.A. and van Santen, E. (1982) Measurement of energy expenditure in humans by doubly labeled water method, *Journal of Applied Physiology*, 53: 955–959.

Schofield, W.N. (1985) Predicting basal metabolic rate, new standards and review of previous work, *Human Nutrition: Clinical Nutrition*, 39, Suppl.1: 5–41.

Schürch, B. and Scrimshaw, N.S (1990)(eds) *Activity, Energy Expenditure and Energy Requirements of Infants and Children*, Proceedings of an International Dietary Energy Consultancy Group workshop, Cambridge, USA, I/D/E/C/G/, Lausanne.

Segal, K.R., Chatr-Artamontri, B. and Guvakov, D. (1994) Validation of a new portable system, *Medicine and Science in Sports and Exercise*, 26: S54.

Spurr, G.B., Dufour, D.L., Reina, J.C. and Haught, T.A. (1997) Daily energy expenditure of women by factorial and heart rate methods, *Medicine and Science in Sports and Exercise*, 29: 1255–1262.

Spurr, G.B., Prentice, A.M., Murgatroyd, P.R., Goldberg, G.R., Reina, J.C. and Christman, N.T. (1988) Energy expenditure using minute-by-minute heart rate recording: comparison with indirect calorimetry, *American Journal of Clinical Nutrition*, 48: 552–559.

Spurr, G.N. (1983) Nutritional status and physical work capacity, *Yearbook of Physical Anthropology*, 26: 1–35.

Thomas, R.B. (1976) Energy flow at high altitude. In Baker, P. T. and Little, M.A. (eds) *Man in the Andes*, Dowden, Hutchinson and Ross, Stroudsburg: 379–404.

Ulijaszek, S.J (1992) Human energetics methods in Biological Anthropology. *Yearbook of Physical Anthropology*, 35: 215–242.

Ulijaszek, S.J. (1995) *Human Energetics in Biological Anthropology*, Cambridge University Press, Cambridge.

Ulijaszek, S.J. and Poraituk, S.P. (1993) Making sago in Papua New Guinea: is it worth the effort?. In Hladik, C.M., Hladik, A., Linares, O.F., Pagézy, H., Semple, A. and Hadley, M. (eds) T*ropical Forests, People and Food: biocultural interactions and applications to development*, Man and the Biosphere series, 13, Unesco, Paris: 271–280.

Varghese, M.A., Saha, P.N. and Atreya, N. (1994) A rapid appraisal of occupational workload from a modified scale of perceived exertion, *Ergonomics*, 37: 485–491.

Wareham, N.J., Hennings, S.J., Prentice, A.M. and Day, N.E. (1997) Feasability of heart rate monitoring to estimate total level and pattern of energy expenditure in a population-based epidemiological study: the Ely young cohort feasibility study 1994–5, *British Journal of Nutrition*, 78: 889–900.

Warwick, P.M., Edmundson, H.M. and Thomson, E.S. (1988) Prediction of energy expenditure: simplified FAO/WHO/UNU factorial method vs. continuous respirometry and habitual energy intake, *American Journal of Clinical Nutrition*, 48: 1188–1196.

Washburn, R.A. and Montoye, H.J. (1986) The assessment of physical activity by questionnaire, *American Journal of Epidemiology*, 123: 563–576.

Wersterterp, K.R. (1999) Physical activity assessment with accelerometers, *International Journal of Obesity and Related Metabolic Disorders*, 23: S45–S49.

# 12. METHODS FOR OBTAINING QUANTITATIVE DATA ON FOOD HABITS IN THE FIRST HALF OF THE TWENTIETH CENTURY

*Isabel González Turmo* and *José Mataix Verdú*

## Hypothesis and Objectives

In 1994, while doing research on Mediterranean food and diet, we faced the need for a method that might enable us to quantify past food habits. More specifically, we wished to embark on an in-depth, comparative study of the cultural and nutritional aspects of food behaviour among the Andalusian population in the past.

Thanks to the surveys carried out by Varela *et al.* (1971), the Instituto Nacional de Estadistica (INE)(1984) and by the Spanish Ministry of Agriculture, Fisheries and Food from 1988 onwards (Ministerio de Agricultura, Pesca y Alimentación 1988, 1991, 1995, 1996, 1998, 1999, 2000), there were enough data over at least a few decades to study change in Andalusian food habits during that period. Subsequently, Dr Mataix Verdú conducted the *Evaluation of the Nutritional Condition of Andalusia*, providing new information on this[1].

A comparison of the results of these surveys revealed that over the last thirty years, the most significant change concerned the percentage composition of the energy intake, which had been noticeably modified by an increase in fats. Proteins had also increased, but the most remarkable alteration was with regard to carbohydrates, more specifically potatoes and bread, which had decreased from 330g to 125g per person and from 380g to 180g per person respectively. Most nutrients, however, kept within values which were similar to those of 1964 (Mataix 1996). These data showed that a relative modification in food habits had taken place. Yet, the change was not so remarkable as to warrant the claim of a new diet and thus, as some nutritional epidemiologists had proposed, of a link between such diet and an increase in cancer, cardio-vascular and degenerative diseases. Rather, we realised that it was necessary to provide more data before the relationship between diet and the general health condition in Andalusia could be pinned down, and that a longer period should be taken into account than the thirty years between 1964 and 1994. However, the earlier diet had not been quantified. All we knew was that it was based on vegetables more than on meat, and that the consumption of bread, pulses and potatoes, all foods which have been cited as part of the 'Mediter-ranean diet', was higher than it is nowadays. González Turmo (1995), there-fore, embarked on a lengthy six-year fieldwork project in order to determine the evolution of Andalusian people's food habits during the twentieth century. However, the quantitative information obtained through this research was exclusively concerned with the present. There were detailed descriptions and qualitative data on the past, but no quantitative information was available.

Thus, our general objective was to analyse and compare the nutrients in regard to three periods (1925–35, 1964 and 1989), placing special emphasis on bread, olive oil and wine. At first, we considered that obtaining data on wine consumption was very important, but we soon had to accept the difficulties in such research. These were partly due to the fact that people, especially women, were reluctant to confess the amount of alcohol they had consumed, and partly due to the fact that men mainly drank alcohol outside of their homes, in bars and pubs. It was, therefore, practically impossible for their wives to inform us on this topic. We were also interested in other factors which did not strictly concern the analysis of nutrients, but were relevant in as far as they concerned food behaviour in general. Among these factors were the siesta, the rhythm and content of meals, which were prepared at the workplace as well as at home, the relationship between diet and the variables related to social status, gender and age, as well as certain culinary aspects.

## Designing the Methods and the Period to be Investigated

When we set out to define our methods, our main problem was to determine what period should be used for the study. In the case of Spain, going back before 1964 meant dealing with the postwar period that followed the 1936–1939 Civil War. Those were years of evident food scarcity and they might have distorted the results of our research. Therefore, since the years between 1936 and 1960 (when food resources at last reached a level of sufficiency) were inappropriate for our aims, we had to go further back in time. The chosen period was that spanning from 1925 to 1935, that is, the decade before the Civil War. Those years were 'normal' in terms of food supplies and it was still poss-ible to find the informants we needed, i.e. elderly, clearheaded women who could remember what they used to eat in their youth. We calculated that the women whose age was between eighty five and ninety five in 1994, had been fifteen to twenty-five years old between 1925 and 1935, which in this society was old enough to have taken part in the purchasing of food and in its preparation in their homes. Later on, we ran into extreme cases like those of daughters who had been entrusted with kitchen chores as early as the age of twelve, because their mothers had had to work outside their home. This, on certain occasions, enabled us to broaden the range of possible informants.

Once the age of women to be surveyed had been defined, the next step was to design a method that might help detect invention or lack of memory. We were aware that we would work with very old people, who might not remember or, even worse, might make up, consciously or not, what they used to eat as young girls. In fact, after the first sample surveys, we realised that most of our informants were women who lived alone or in an old people's home. They were so eager to talk and to be listened to that they would have answered the interviewer, even if they remembered nothing about what was being asked. It was, therefore, necessary to find a way of retrieving the old people's genuine recollections, separating them from what was being invented or inaccurately 'remembered'.

The method consisted of gathering the same information in three different records, in order to verify later the concordance of the data collected. In the first place we collected data from informants whom we termed 'privileged' because they were in a privileged position to provide helpful information, i.e. they were old enough in the decade between 1925 and 1935 to have already been working as butchers, bakers, fishermen, dairymaids, etc. It is worth remembering that in those days children started to work or to help their families from a young age.

González Turmo's previous research (1995) on Andalusian food habits in the twentieth century had shown that the food quantities which were then purchased never varied. A family would buy the same amount of bread or meat from one to three times a week. The same was true of olive oil. Thus, we presumed that bakers and butchers would be able to remember quite clearly the daily quantity of bread consumed by a family of six or ten members, or the quantity of meat used in stews, which were always likely to be the same. The data obtained from these privileged informants in each place we studied would serve as a starting point for subsequent interviews with the elderly women. So, for example, if the quantity of meat the women said they used to eat diverged significantly from the information obtained previously, we deduced that their memory was failing or that they were referring to a later period or that they were confused in some other way. Our conclusion, nevertheless, was that members of the middle class ate *cocido* (a stew made with pulses, meat and pork sausages) daily, but most of the population made do with *puchero* (this is the name of the cooking pot and is a humbler version of *cocido*) only once a week.

After interviewing our privileged informants we surveyed the elderly women using two different registers: one recorded what they used to eat, the other what they used to buy or produce.

The first record showed the weekly consumption as deduced from the various meals of the day, at home as well as at the workplace, and the enquiry included every member of the domestic group. Two seasons, winter and summer, were considered. Thus, we were able to determine how many times a week a certain stew was consumed. We inquired about the recipe, quantities and weight of its ingredients and seasoning, as well as about timetables and characteristics regarding commensality. A problem which we had to face constantly during the surveys was the relative ease with which our informants' discourse skipped to later periods, especially to the postwar years when hunger would build up as an indelible memory.

The second record was for information gathered on purchases of each of the various food groups. The interviewees could answer with daily, weekly or monthly quantities, depending on the frequency with which a given food was usually bought. So, for example, bread was purchased daily and olive oil monthly. We thus facilitated the women´s recollection of facts. Data were gathered on the following foodstuffs: bread, fruit and vegetables, dairy products and eggs, olives, oil and fats, meat, fish, drinks and products hunted or gathered.

First we asked what the origin of each food was. We took into account the food type and quantity (depending on the season) and whether it had been purchased, produced for their own consumption, bartered or received as a gift. Secondly, we inquired about frequency and thirdly, about the cooking methods used for the elaboration of such food.

This technique allowed us to discard many surveys before they were completed and, in the worst of cases, after their completion. Data concerning purchase and consumption, at least as far as the main food groups were concerned, had necessarily to square up. We demanded reliability in the first place for foodstuffs like bread, oil and meat, and in the second place for pulses, potatoes, dairy products, eggs, fish and wine. As for fruit and vegetables, however, we knew that the margin of error was very broad, since in many cases these foods were cultivated by the interviewees themselves and it was impossible to convert the quantities provided by our informants (baskets, hampers, etc.) to the metric system.

If the data relating to the purchasing of the first food group did not agree relatively well with those related to consumption that case study was discarded. This implied a great deal of work because only one third of the surveys turned out to be useful for our research. Yet, those which fulfilled the demanded degree of reliability could be included with absolute confidence.

## Selection of Interviewers and Informants, and Phases of the Research

In order to try out our methodology, we chose Conil, a place on the southern limits of Andalusia, very close to the Straits of Gibraltar which separate Europe from Africa. We worked with six privileged informants and eight elderly women. This allowed us to make some modifications and define the quantities described by our informants. Since they used handfuls, breakfast mugs, plates, glasses, etc., instead of the metric system, we had to weigh such quantities with utensils belonging to the period under consideration, in order to make sure that the quantity calculated today was the same as that of the period in question. Rafael Toledo, who was our collaborator in the project, took the trouble to weigh the quantities that appeared time and again: a handful of chickpeas or rice, a cup of milk, a glass of wine, a 'fist-like' piece of bread, etc. Afterwards, we could provide the interviewers with a table of measures, which enabled them to note down, for example, the quantity of chickpeas in grams, every time the informant referred to a handful of chickpeas.

The next step was to select the interviewers, the places and the informants. The interviewers were mainly students doing their PhD in the Anthropology of Food, or collaborators of Dr Mataix Verdú[2]. In total eighteen[3] worked on the research in thirteen locations[4]. We tried to cover the whole geography of Andalusia, taking into account the distribution of our working locations, but, in the end, most of the locations obtained for the research turned out to be in western Andalusia.

Interviewers were trained in three alternate years. In addition to explaining and debating the methodology, much emphasis was placed on the fact that students should avoid influencing answers, a particularly delicate issue when it comes to working with elderly people, since they do not usually trust their own memory and are all too ready to appropriate the interviewers' suggestions. Stress was also put on the need for a description of the mentioned foods, since we had already experienced frequent cases of homonymy and synonymy in Andalusia concerning bread, fruit and vegetables.

Our informants were elderly women, not all of them suited to the objectives of our investigation. Our main interest lay in understanding the past food habits of the majority of the population, not those of the elite. Therefore, we only worked with women belonging to the working class, peasantry, or families of retailers and artisans. Another requirement for the research was that the informants' families must have lived in the chosen place for at least two generations and that they had not migrated there during the years which were being studied.

The work done during those years, as a result of the postgraduate courses, was repeated in other Andalusian locations in 1999 and 2000, by graduates María del Mar Pérez López and Cristina Álvarez Rey[5]. The results of these latest surveys will, as we receive them, be processed by Isabela Justo, who had processed the previous ones. The final results are not yet available. The collection of data comes to an end with these last surveys, since most of the women who may have cooked between 1925 and 1935 have already died. Without their assistance it would have been impossible to record recollections which were about to disappear and which were crucial to our knowledge of the past food habits of Andalusians.

## Conclusion

Information about the past sought through interviews with elderly subjects needs to be treated with caution, and efforts should be made to check the data given against some other types of information. This is as true in regard to food consumption and habits as it is in regard to any other topic. In this chapter methods used to judge the validity of memories and reminiscences about food consumption in a period sixty to seventy years earlier in Andalusia are clearly described. Three approaches were used and only data which were shown to be concordant in all three approaches could be trusted. The fact that information given by some elderly informants did not agree well with the other methods of study demonstrates the need for researchers to find these different ways to check oral data. As discussed in other chapters in this volume, this can also be the case for information on contemporary food habits.

## Acknowledgements

The authors wish to express their satisfaction with and gratitude to all those who have taken part in this project as respondents and as interviewers. The support of the Andalusian Health Council is acknowledged.

## Notes

1. This research was supported by the Andalusian Health Council. Dr. Mataix was also adviser for the investigations carried out in the Basque country (1992), Catalunya (1994) and Galicia (1993).
2. The former were students attending the doctoral course, *Food systems and Cultural Identity*, which Dr González Turmo has been teaching since 1994. The latter were students attending the *Course for Specialists in Nutrition and Dietetics* at the Andalusian Institute of Nutrtiion, supervised by Dr Mataix Verdú.
3. The students' names were: Berraquero García, I., Cansinar Bernal, R., Díaz González, M.,Durán Salado, Mª I., García Díaz, A., Guerra Martín, Mª D., Heredia Sancho, J. M., Jiménez Aguado, M., Jiménez de León, E., Laliena Sanz, A.C., Martínez Keina, J.M., Miranda Ruiz de Lacanal, C., Montero Fernández, C., Román Oliver, J., Ruiz Cerezuela, D., Ruíz Morales, F. C., Salas, R., Toledo, R.. González Turmo, I. worked in Conil (Cádiz) and Ronda (Málaga).
4. The locations were: Alcalá de Guadaira (Sevilla), Camas (Sevilla), Castilleja de la Cuesta (Sevilla), Conil (Cádiz), Dos Hermanas (Sevilla), Guadiz (Granada), Higuera de la Sierra (Huelva), María (Almería), Montellano (Sevilla), Ronda (Málaga), Sanlúcar de Barrameda (Cádiz), Sevilla, Utrera (Sevilla).
5. These locations were: Alcalar la Real (Jaen), Baena (Córdoba), Córdoba, Loja (Granada), Mojacar (Almería), Montefrío (Granada), Periana (Málaga).

# References

González Turmo, I. (1995) *Comida de rico, comida de pobre. La transformación de los hábitos alimenticios en el Occidente andaluz, S XX,* Universidad de Sevilla Press, Seville, (2nd Edition in 1997).

Instituto Nacional de Estadística (1984) *El consumo de alimentos, bebidas y tabacos en cantidades físicas (1980/81),* Encuesta de presupuestos familiares, Madrid.

Mataix, J. (1996) Evolución de la dieta española en la segunda mitad del siglo XX. In González Turmo, I. and Romero de Solís, P. (eds) *Antropología de la Alimentación: nuevos ensayos sobre la Dieta Mediterránea,* Universidad de Sevilla Press, Seville: 65–76.

Ministerio de Agricultura, Pesca y Alimentación (1988) *Consumo alimentario en España 1987,* Dirección General de Política Alimentaria, Madrid.

Ministerio de Agricultura, Pesca y Alimentación (1991) *Consumo alimentario en España 1990,* Dirección General de Política Alimentaria, Madrid.

Ministerio de Agricultura, Pesca y Alimentación (1995) *Consumo alimentario en España 1994,* Dirección General de Política Alimentaria, Madrid.

Ministerio de Agricultura, Pesca y Alimentación (1996*) Consumo alimentario en España 1995,* Dirección General de Política Alimentaria, Madrid.

Ministerio de Agricultura, Pesca y Alimentación (1998*) Consumo alimentario en España 1998,* Dirección General de Política Alimentaria, Madrid.

Ministerio de Agricultura, Pesca y Alimentación (1999*) Consumo alimentario en España 1999,* Dirección General de Política Alimentaria, Madrid.

Ministerio de Agricultura, Pesca y Alimentación (2000) *Consumo alimentario en España 2000,* Dirección General de Política Alimentaria, Madrid.

Varela, G., García, D. and Moreiras, O. (1971) La *nutrición de los españoles: diagnóstico y recomendaciones,* Estudios del Instituto de Desarrollo Económico, Madrid.

# 13. RECONSTRUCTING DIETS FOR COMPENSATION FOR NUCLEAR TESTING IN RONGELAP, MARSHALL ISLANDS

*Nancy J. Pollock*

In order to reconstruct a diet the anthropologist must rely on a number of sources of information which comprise what Geertz (1993) has termed 'the web of culture'. The place of food in culture has slowly gained recognition from Richards' (1939) studies to more recent analyses (e.g. Lupton 1996). Diet may be assessed from a biological approach to intake/output or from an ecological approach showing uses of local foods, or from a broad social anthropological approach that considers food as an essential component of social life (Pollock 1992). Food, then, is circumscribed by cultural bounds that contribute to the unique identity of a community. Reconstruction of a diet must draw upon written accounts of a society's past, plant inventories, historical settings, and personal knowledge of community members. Where that reconstruction aims to account for health outcomes, as in the case discussed here, then the anthropologist must collaborate with health physicists to construct a broader picture than either specialist alone could provide. This chapter is about how an anthropologist was involved in a cross-disciplinary study of dietary reconstruction. Of necessity some ethnographic details are included.

The people concerned in this case study lived until 1985 on one atoll in the northern Marshalls, in the central Pacific (Map, see Figure 13.1). These Rongelap people had been exposed to radioactive fallout from a nuclear bomb test on Bikini, an atoll some 200 miles to the west. The test, code-named Bravo, was part of a United States military defence strategy of nuclear preparedness during the Cold War. On 1 March, 1954, Bravo sent a cloud of radioactive material into the upper atmosphere that travelled eastward to land on Rongelap and other atolls. The people living on Rongelap at that time have subsequently suffered many serious health problems. These include cancer of the

*Figure 13.1*   Map of Pacific Ocean showing Marshall Islands

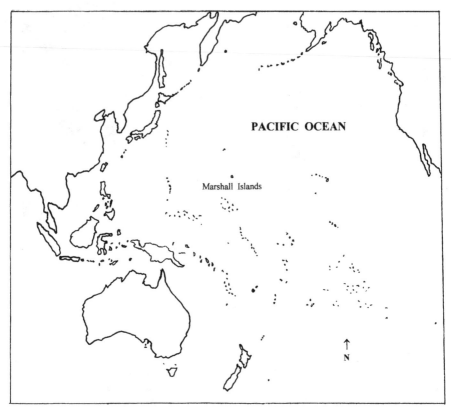

goitre, and cancers of many other parts of their body; one young man, aged nineteen, died of leukaemia in 1972. The health problems resulted from the people continuing to live on land that remained highly radioactive and eating contaminated food. United States health teams filed annual reports that stated that no serious health problems were occurring. Both ingested radiation and background radiation continued until 1985, when the people moved themselves off Rongelap to take up residence on a nearby uncontaminated atoll (see Pollock 2001 for details).

Since no record was kept in the 1950s and 1960s of what these people were eating, my own detailed recording of the diets of people living on an atoll 150 miles to the south of Rongelap (Pollock 1970) has formed one base for the reconstruction exercise. That study on Namu atoll included both dietary and social information, which turned out to be important for the health physicists engaged in this exercise.

In this chapter I will discuss four sets of factors that proved useful in the reconstruction of the diet of the Rongelap people: dietary factors, social factors, health factors and the need for cross-disciplinary liaison and cooperation between different specialists. The aim was to assess the impact of ingested radiation on their bodies, for example resulting in cancers, particularly of the goitre. A dietary record from fifty years ago had to be reconstructed, amplified by social factors and addressing health outcomes, all set within a framework of the period between 1954 and the present. A second dimension required construction of a diet for the future once radiation is cleared from the Rongelap atoll. The dietary record from the past and the projected diet for the peoples' return to Rongelap formed part of their claim for compensation from the United States for the effects of fallout from the nuclear testing programme in the 1950s. Yet, the literature on dietary recall suggests that two days is the maximum time over which to expect reasonably accurate data from informants (Mead 1945, Hegsted 1985). So, attempting to reconstruct dietary information over a fifty-year period requires a combination of skills. When that dietary information is needed to assess health problems due to radiation exposure, the anthropologist can provide ethnographic information to botanists about local foods, and to health physicists about living habits that have contributed to health problems. This combination of specialist knowledge was required by lawyers in order to argue the case for compensation to this population from the United States government (Nuclear Claims Tribunal 2001). The differences between the anthropologist's data and that used by health physicists is set out for each category below.

A local food only diet was the main focus of attention, though imported foods, particularly rice, had to be incorporated into the final analysis. Local foods were important not only in terms of type and frequency of consumption, but also in terms of their radioactive content. A major difficulty has been that knowledge of the effects of radiation and radioactive substances on the human body has changed dramatically over the past fifty years. In the 1950s information about health hazards from ingested radioactive foods was not as sophisticated as it is today. Furthermore, a political agenda of secrecy surrounding all nuclear testing activities and the communities involved exacerbated the difficulties of this exercise (Pringle and Spigelman 1982).

## Dietary Records

Anthropologists have become more meticulous about recording dietary information over the last ten to fifteen years. Any dietary record consists of several components, depending on the orientation of the researcher. For the anthropologist the broad picture is important as a background for interpreting dietary variation, as well as the specifics of food use in the cultural setting. Previously, foods eaten were recorded only as part of the economic activity of a society, with the focus mainly on the production of food rather than on its consumption. So foods cooked and eaten together, amounts eaten, local reasons for selecting food, meal structures and the social relationships involved in sharing food tended to be given less attention.

Nutritionists generally recorded individual foods and their chemical content in order to construct a nutritional base either for individuals or for a population. Their profile of caloric intake and expenditure and the contributions of vitamins and minerals to the well-being of the people would lead to an evaluation of the nutritional adequacy of that diet, based on western Recommended Dietary Allowances, as defined by the World Health Organisation. Nuclear physicists also tend to concentrate on individual foods, omitting to consider the social context. Frequently, these analyses overlooked the symbolic importance of food, and its fundamental significance in the Pacific within an ethic of sharing and generosity. Such an omission ignored the importance of diet as an integral part of total social well-being, as is discussed in the next section.

## Research Methods used for the Reconstruction of the Rongelap Diet

A food inventory was the first step. The list of foods used on Rongelap and their availability at different times during the year was compiled from my own fieldwork and from botanical information. In addition combinations of foods always eaten together, such as rice and coconut cream, were recorded. Methods of cooking were also important information as they indicated the handling of local fuel wood, mainly coconut husks, and that also entailed radiation exposure. Also the times that food was consumed (what we call 'meals' in English) give an indication not only of the amount of food consumed but also of the expected rhythm of daily life. An important distinction for this study was that between foods obtained locally and those imported, since local foods were deemed to be the source of ingested radioactivity.

A basic list of foods available in the northern Marshalls, detailed by Pollock (1992) was amplified by written records from Rongelap dating from the 1950s and 1960s in order to include food sources referred to by visitors. Local foods in the Marshall Islands are limited by the ecology of atolls, so both coralline soils and rainfall are important determinants. Also one had to bear in mind that some foods were seasonal or were consumed only on particular occasions, such as at feasts. Furthermore, one had to consider what was eaten fresh and what was fermented.

Since the 1950s local foods had been increasingly added to by purchased foods, bought off trading ships. With rapid population growth every atoll has come to rely on purchasing foods from visiting trade ships in order to supplement local foods. From the 1960s to the present, these imports have consisted of four main items: rice, flour, tea and sugar, with some fat (Crisco) and an occasional case of canned fish or meat. I have detailed records of food intake, and have noted that the basic Marshallese diet has changed very little for outer island people over the twenty-five years that I have been working there (Pollock 1995).

The concept of a meal had to be introduced to refer to the major eating event of the day (Pollock 2001). This meal is eaten once a day, in the evening, with leftovers consumed the next morning. Some households may cook some rice for the children for a midday meal. Studying the structure and content of these eating events was important for calculating the total amounts of any person's daily intake of radioactive substances, and estimating any points of variation over an annual cycle. A total food record must include feasts for the variation they offer to the daily diet. In the Marshalls feasts were notable for including a wider range of foodstuffs than that in daily household fare. Sunday food is a mini-feast in the sense that fishermen of the household attempt to provide enough fish for everyone, and women make special puddings.

Thus an anthropological record of a seven day diet for selected times during the year cycle is more likely to include these special food events than a nutritionist's one or two day diet record (see also Henry and Macbeth this volume). By recording seven day's consumption every month for ten out of fifteen months of fieldwork, I was able to note the importance of the seasonality of breadfruit and pandanus in their contribution to the diet, and also the variability over the seasons in the amount of fish available. Diet also varied according to the arrival of a trading ship, and these arrivals were highly erratic due to disruptions by United States nuclear testing activity over Kwajalein and medical evacuations. Since those ships bought copra, they were the sole source of cash for households, as well as the islanders' only means of obtaining additional food supplies.

## Cooperation with Nuclear Physicists

The nuclear physicists were faced with two tasks: (1) to estimate the dosage of radiation the Rongelap people had ingested and absorbed during the twenty-eight years they had remained on their island; and (2) to calculate the likely levels of radiation present in Rongelap plants and soils after clean-up for the purpose of developing a diet for the future that would meet the safety levels for radiation uptake today. The second exercise was more contentious because there remain so many unknowns in the Pacific diet (see Neel *et al.* 1994). The target set by the Rehabilitation Committee for Rongelap people was a dosage of not more than 100 rem, the unit rate of absorption of radioactivity (see Siwatibau and Williams 1985 for a definition of rem and other nuclear radiation terms, also briefly introduced below). That target level is based both on foods likely to be ingested on their return, and also on any residual background radiation.

Findings of an excess prevalence of thyroid nodules in the Marshallese population have resulted in several studies of the doses of radiation these people received as a result of fallout from Bravo and other United States test series in the 1950s (Hamilton *et al.* 1987, Musolino *et al.* 1997). Those data are based mainly on external exposure, rather than from ingested foods. In hindsight, the likely exposure 168 hours after fallout (on 1 March, 1954) was calculated and multiplied by the 'decay corrected thyroid absorbed dose' (Musolino *et al.* 1997: 655). It was found that high thyroid absorption doses had occurred in Rongelap and other northern Marshall Islands, so that 'a systematic medical survey for thyroid disease should be conducted, and ... a more definitive dose reconstruction should be made for all the populated atolls and islands in the Northern Marshalls' (Musolino *et al.* 1997: 651).

Individual local foods had been analysed by the National Radiation Laboratory in Majuro to reveal the main isotopes present after radiation (Simon 1992). These included Iodine 131, Strontium 90, Carbon 14, Plutonium 239 and Cesium 137. Iodine 131 was particularly notorious because it concentrates in the thyroid, and could thus account for the high rates of thyroid cancer in the Rongelap population. Strontium 90 is pernicious because of its slow rate of decay.

Much debate had occurred over the fifty years since the first atomic bomb explosions as to what were 'safe' levels for daily and annual exposure to radiation. Two terms are used for measurements in general discussion of radiation levels: (1) the 'rad', for radiation absorbed dose, which measures the actual radiation absorbed by the object being penetrated; and (2) the 'rem', for roentgen equivalent man, which is used for biological damage caused by radiation. One thousandth of a 'rem', or 'millirem', is the unit for measuring safe levels of radiation (Pringle and Spigelman 1982:501, Siwatibau and Williams 1985). An annual intake of 100 rem has been set as the basic standard which cleanup must attain, according to a Memorandum of Understanding between the Rongelap people and the United States government (Nuclear Claims Tribunal 2001).

Such information was hard to obtain in the 1950s and 1960s. It remains a matter of speculation as to whether scientists knew some of the likely outcomes of ingested radiation, or were experimenting on the effects on human bodies, by using the Rongelap population as 'guinea pigs' (Special Joint Committee report 1973). The intense secrecy surrounding these military tests in the 1950s and 1960s resulted in any discussions being limited only to those involved, and under strict military confidentiality. Wider discussion has been forthcoming only after records were declassified in 1979. Criticism and assessment of those records have begun to emerge (e.g. Pringle and Spigelman 1982), and it is an aspect of such cross-disciplinary research that attempts should be made to follow up all possible reports and written records.

## Dietary Scenarios

In discussions leading up to the Compensation hearings (November 2001, and August 2000), a so-called 'local diet' was the main focus for assessing radiation dose rates. The health physicists' food inventory that had been drawn up in the

United States (Naidu and Greenhouse 1980) was heavily criticised by the National Research Council panel for methodological issues (Neel *et al.* 1994: 41–51). It did not cover the full annual cycle, it lacked information on informants' living conditions, interviewers were not experienced nutritionists or dieticians or familiar with local foods, etc. As a result the 1980 inventory included foods rarely used in the Marshall Islands, e.g. meat and eggs, which were rarely available, and the list was devised from current usage, rather than from reconstructed usage in the 1950s and 1960s. A revised list had to be negotiated, and the social dimensions had to be included in the health physicists' calculations.

For the Compensation hearings, three dietary scenarios, drawn from the Neel *et al.* report (1994) were used as the basis for calculating the future diet. A 'local only diet' was contrasted with a diet of 'imported food only', while a third scenario consisted of mixed imported and local foods. The purists wanted the calculations to focus on the Rongelap people eating only their local foods when they return. But this point was overturned by persuasive arguments that the plants will take a long time to become re-established and bear fruits after the land has been successfully cleared of all radioactive material – and that could be some twenty years in the future, since clearing only commenced in 2001. In addition, I argued that the Rongelap people, like other Marshallese, have been using rice as a significant component of their diet for fifty years, and so they are not likely to give it up even if a bounty of local food were a feasible scenario. So, the final calculations aimed to establish a scenario of local only food with twenty-five percent imported food/rice component.

## Social Factors

Any assessment of radiation exposure had to place eating habits, both in the past and in the future, in their cultural context, and this was exemplified in this multidisciplinary study.

Land and the sea are the sources of all local foods. Thus land rights that give households access to these resources need to be considered. Households are located on sites handed down in the matrilineal line, and thus are composed of women, their children and husbands, and their mother. Households thus consist of several nuclear families of sisters. They share sleeping accommodation, a common cooking place, and toilet facilities. Food is cooked by the younger women on a roster basis, although women should not cook for their husbands when they are menstruating. Food is usually eaten in nuclear family groups sitting outside, except in bad weather.

Food is gathered rather than dug up. As the tree crops ripen, they are harvested by household members. Women may gather these on their household sites or other lands to which they have rights. Men gather on their mother's, and thus also their sisters', lands. Attention to his mother's needs is a first call on a man's labour, but he must also assist with provisioning his household of residence, that is that of his wife and children. Similarly any fish he catches is divided between his mother and sisters' household, and his wife and children's household.

Keeping track of who shares in any household's food supply requires close recording on a regular basis. Children may eat at any one of several households where they have relatives. A child may eat and sleep with any of his or her mother's sisters' children, or with households related to the father. A nuclear family within a household is likely to move several times during any one year period of observation, both within the atoll or off island to another atoll, or to spend time in Majuro or Ebeye, the two urban centres.

Calculating population size on Rongelap was a major concern in assessing diets and those affected by radiation. Rapid population growth on atolls of the Marshalls has led to some out-migration as well as increasing pressure on local food resources. Those who return from a district centre are likely to bring some canned food, and other goods such as rice and flour. The large cohort of people under twenty-five years of age has not only placed pressure on local food resources, but they have developed a desire for quick, tasty, varied and western-style foods, not easily obtained on the outer islands. So, food is one reason given for moving elsewhere.

Imported food is seen as desirable for a variety of reasons. But the money to purchase it is hard to come by. On outer islands, such as Rongelap itself, copra, the dried 'meat' of coconut, has been the only source of cash for the last forty years. Rongelap people have received some small pay-outs from the United States government for 'rent' of their atoll, and for health problems and some of that money has been used to buy imported food on a regular basis. As coconut trees were limited in number on Rongelap, copra realised only small cash sums.

Imported food has thus become more necessary over the last fifty years. Food preferences have changed. Rice is quick and easy to cook, whereas breadfruit must be scraped in the coals, and arrowroot must be carefully leached before the starch is available. Canned food tastes good, but is costly so the amount each person on an outer island receives is limited to about 30 to 50 grams very irregularly. Fishing thus provides a vital supplement to the diet.

Amounts eaten by individuals of various ages provide important information for researchers reconstructing diets. Practices influencing amounts of food accessible to various ages, and to each gender are very culturally specific. The amounts actually eaten, as distinct from estimated intake, can vary with the health and well-being of the individuals involved. Thus a daily record of a household's consumption must account for these variations (e.g. x was sick with 'flu', y was staying at r's household, etc.). Also, it is important to record any food that is discarded, usually to pigs and chickens, particularly when assessing diet and health concerns.

Year round variability in food supply is an important part of the record. A period of scarcity can reduce the overall average caloric intake considerably, and may increase the consumption of foods high in radioactive isotopes, for example coconut. For the population of Namu in the northern Marshalls my figures of an average of 1900 calories per day, with no vegetables, calculated over a fifteen month period were deemed unacceptable by nutritionists. Yet women lactated profusely on what nutritionists would claim to be a 'poor' diet. Since women are either pregnant or lactating for most of their reproductive life, I argue that they have adapted their total life style to enable them and their children to survive, with some losses. Reproductive losses due to radio-activity, e.g. still births of malformed foetuses, hydatidiform cysts, etc., were at first denied by the Nuclear Claims Tribunal, but recently have been included for compensation. This identifies a significant difference in conclusions between the short term studies by visiting nutritionists and the longer term, holistic observations by an anthropologist.

## Liaison with Health Physicists

The health physicists did not initially have access to many of these social factors, even though the National Research Council report (Neel *et al.* 1994) had underlined their importance. The figures calculated for the dietary scenarios discussed above applied only to the 'average' adult for one day's intake over a year. No special calculations were made for children (and children have been severely affected by radiation exposure). Household composition was not considered. Nor were feasts and seasonal variability taken into account. Initial calculations had placed higher values on the fish than on the starch food, as they presumed (from western food habits) that the protein sector was more important than the starch sector of the diet. Their calculations were thus not based on locally observed dietary practices. Work practices were presumed rather than based on ethnographic information.

One danger in reconstructing both past and future diets for the Rongelap people is that the range and amounts of food are so limited that any dosage of ingested radiation may be magnified significantly if one or other local food is not available. An average figure may thus be a significant miscalculation. Furthermore, no attempt was made to estimate radiation levels in rice, an imported food, which may sit for a month or more in sacks on the ground that contained significant levels of radiation.

Fish continues to be a source of speculation for the diets reconstructed by the health physicists. They argue that since fish introduced inorganic iodide into the diet, the traditional diet that included seafood was sufficient to prevent endemic goitre. Thus they are considering whether dietary iodide would be sufficient to meet the needs for new iodide to replace obligatory losses in the urine and sweat. However, the broader question is how much fish, over the yearly cycle, is necessary to provide this prevention against goitre? These estimates of radioactive iodine in the Bravo fallout diet, which went to the thyroid and caused subsequent damage, may result in $US200 million on this question alone (HC personal communication).

The Rongelap people constantly expressed concern about the safety of the fish, which they were eating from their lagoon. They were told that they did not carry any radioactivity, but today that judgement is being questioned. New questions keep emerging that the health physicists realise require answers, rather than assumptions from their own social background to dietary practices. The role of the anthropologist is likely to be significant in the multidisciplinary attempts to answer these questions.

## Importance of the Anthropologist's Participant Observation

The anthropologist can provide useful information from longer term observations, while the casual visitor, such as a health physicist, may not grasp the significance, for example, of the movement of foods between households. Food in any of the Pacific islands is a 'total social fact'. It is both a material entity that has one set of values and a strong symbol with many wider values. Generosity with food is an accepted principle, no matter how much or how little is available. This generosity leads to ongoing exchanges of food between households, both on and off the island, and to gifts to visitors and to chiefs. Food offered to a person passing the house is a significant call on any household's supplies, but may not be recalled.

The social context of food was not recorded by the Brookhaven National Laboratory (BNL) staff who visited Rongelap annually from 1957 to 1980. Even though studying the health of the people, they did not (apparently) record what those people were eating, let alone any other features of food that might have associated food with the intake of radiation. However, the current health physicists have come to recognise its importance in reconstructing dosages of background radiation and the relevance of liaison with an anthropologist. An anthropologist can provide ethnographic details about food, that food is seldom wasted, that gifts and exchange are important, that spare fish may be salted and dried, etc., which in turn may be relevant to the reconstruction of likely sources of radiation. For example, plans by United States officials to remediate/clean only the village areas have overlooked the importance of fishing activities for men, and families who picnic and visit outer islets for a week or two at a time. If those outer islets are still 'hot' with radiation, then they will need to be cleaned and/or people warned of the dangers to their health by visiting them.

An anthropologist can confirm that the Rongelap people have observed their own health deteriorating over the last forty years. Throughout the BNL team's monitoring of their health, the people were concerned that the team kept returning and yet reporting that the people were not experiencing any serious health problems. Their food became a target of suspicion. As they asked more specialists they learned a lot about the effects of ingested radiation, and thus their food has fallen under a cloud of suspicion (see Siwatibau and Williams 1985).

## Conclusions

The methods outlined here for dietary reconstruction of a particular case have a certain level of generality. A dietary inventory is basic to any dietary reconstruction. It should include the source of production or market of each food. The social setting in which foods are consumed must also be outlined, that outline tailored to the particular case in point. Here that social setting is integral to understanding the calculations of both ingested and background radiation that has led to the health problems. Other observations and changes that affect the diet must also be noted.

Dietary reconstruction by the anthropologist requires special methods drawn from a number of knowledge areas. Oral history, environmental study, and nutrition or medical history, as well as traditional anthropological approaches, provide useful indicators as to how to manage the exercise. Those techniques will need to be adjusted to the particular aims of each exercise. At the same time, the anthropologist may need to address questions posed by health researchers, or any other specialists whose work impinges on the question to hand. Also, the anthropologists contribute questions of their own to the wider debate.

In the case study discussed here, the aim was both to contribute to understanding the health problems the Rongelap people had suffered from ingesting radioactive substances over a thirty year period, as well as to calculate future safety levels of ingested radioactivity after the atoll is cleaned up. The people themselves are very sceptical about the safety level of radioactivity that any outside group of scientists may propose. They expect to be able to eat their own local foods, as the land is replanted, as well as to continue to use imported foods, such as rice and flour and canned goods. But the reality may be that they will eat only imported food because local plants are slow regenerating.

A major difference between the perspective of the anthropologist and that of the health physicist or the nutritionist is that the former approaches these considerations from a community perspective, while the latters' major concern is with individual levels of ingestion. This is a major divergence of approaches. Negotiation can be tedious, but rewarding. Variation versus a normative picture is another point of debate.

A major philosophical concern is the rapid change in ideas that all these disciplines have experienced over the last twenty or thirty years. As nutritional concerns have changed between the 1960s and the present time, so anthropological concerns are also vastly different today. These changes in attitudes need to be realised as they have a marked effect on outcomes. This was certainly true in trying to reconstruct levels of radioactivity that have caused such harm to the health of the Rongelap people. If the new approach of reconstruction can assist them in living safer lives in the future, then it has been doubly worthwhile.

# References

Geertz, C. (1993) *The Interpretation of Cultures,* Fontana Press, London.

Hamilton, T.E., van Belle, G. and LoGerfo, J.P. (1987) Thyroid neoplasia in Marshall Islanders exposed to nuclear fallout, *Journal of the American Medical Association,* 258: 629–636.

Hegsted, D. (1985) Nutrition: the changing scene, *Nutrition Reviews,* 43(12): 347–367.

Lupton, D. (1996) *Food, the Body and the Self,* Sage Publications, London.

Mead, M. (1945) *Manual for the Study of Food Habits,* National Research Council, Washington.

Musolino, S.V., Greenhouse, A. and Hull, A.P. (1997) An estimate by two methods of thyroid absorbed doses due to Bravo fallout in several northern Marshall Islands, *Health Physics,* 73(4), 651–662.

Naidu, J.R. and Greenhouse, A. (1980) *Marshall Islands: a study of diet and living patterns,* Brookhaven National Laboratory Technical Document No. 51313, Brookhaven.National Laboratory, Upton, New York.

Neel, J. , Zimbrick, J. and Taylor, D. (1994) *Radiological Assessments for Resettlement of Rongelap in the Republic of the Marshall Islands,* National Academy Press, Washington

Nuclear Claims Tribunal (2001) *Rongelap Hearings,* Website: www.nctamar.com.

Pollock, N.J. (1970) *Breadfruit and Breadwinning on Namu, a Marshallese atoll,* Ph.D thesis, Department of Anthropology, University of Hawaii.

Pollock, N.J. (1992) *These Roots Remain,* The Institute for Polynesian Studies, and University of Hawaii Press, Hawaii.

Pollock, N.J. (1995) Namu atoll revisited: a follow up study of 25 years of resource use, *Atoll Research Bulletin,* No. 441.

Pollock, N.J. (2001) The Marshall Islanders. In Fitzpatrick, J. (ed.) *Endangered Peoples of Oceania: struggles to survive and thrive,* Greenwood Press, Westport, Connecticut.

Pringle, P. and Spigelman, J. (1982) *The Nuclear Barons,* Michael Joseph, London.

Richards, A. (1939) *Hunger and Work amongst the Bemba of Northern Rhodesia,* Oxford University Press, London.

Simon, S. (1992) *Rongelap Atoll Resettlement Project,* Technical Planning Document for Radiological Monitoring Activities, National Radiation Laboratory, Majuro, Marshall Islands.

Siwatibau, S. and Williams, D. (1985) *A Call to a New Exodus: an anti-nuclear primer for Pacific People,* Pacific Conference of Churches, Suva.

Special Joint Committee concerning Rongelap and Utirik Atolls (1973) *A Report on Rongelap and Utirik to the Congress of Micronesia: medical aspects of the incident of March 1, 1954.* Public Law# 4C-33, (Manuscript in Hancock Library of the Australian National University, Canberra, Australia).

# 14. FOOD, CULTURE, POLITICAL AND ECONOMIC IDENTITY
## REVITALISING THE FOOD-SYSTEMS PERSPECTIVE IN THE STUDY OF FOOD-BASED IDENTITY

*Ellen Messer*

## Introduction

Food is a basic concern for all human societies, and reflecting on this basic concern, anthropologists have long been interested in human diets. From a food-systems perspective, anthropologists have studied (a) the ecological and market availability of foods, (b) the sociocultural classifications of foods as 'edible' or 'inedible', the rankings of 'preferred' or 'less preferred' foods, and rules for distribution, and (c) the nutritional and medical consequences of particular cultural consumption patterns, including patterns of food sharing. We have also explored from sociological, psychological, ecological, and nutritional perspectives how diets and humans have evolved, and the biocultural significance of food in construction of sociocultural identities. The traditional proverbs, 'Tell me what you eat and I'll tell you who you are' (from the French) and 'You are what you eat' (from the German) point to some more general issues connecting food to cultural identity: the relationships of human populations or social groups to their environment; the symbolic construction of cultures; the social relations and social structures that constitute and, in identifiable times and places, embody social change (Messer 1984). Anthropologists explicitly bring to this topic of 'identity' combinations of biological and sociocultural perspectives that can illuminate the local implications of globalisation, specifically of the global circulation of foodstuffs, that involve interrelated processes of social, dietary and culinary change.

Several recent articles and volumes organised by American anthropologists have attempted to make food studies, or the study of food and identity, a major theme in postmodern and experimental anthropology. Positively, these studies tend to be multilevelled cultural analyses, which consider the meanings of the food, including the manner of its preparation and consumption, from multiple cultural perspectives. James Watson's edited volume (1997) explores the meaning of fast food, hamburger-and-fries establishments in multiple Asian settings. He and the contributors to his book consider how people in different places and populations (Beijing, Japan, Taipei, Hong Kong and Seoul) take the generic fast-food restaurant and make it their own, both by adding some locally desirable ingredients or dishes or, alternatively, by making the transnational food emporia serve some cultural goal. Examples of cultural goals might be that of providing a safe meeting place for grandmother and grandchild, for young teens with their peers, and/or for otherwise housebound wives who may want to get out and perhaps rebel against their subservient roles, or simply that of providing a bright and sanitary place (with clean bathrooms) to eat out. Whether or not these Asian national societies have managed to coopt food globalisation and avoid McDonaldisation, domination and culinary deculturalisation, such 'localisation of the globalisation' studies appear incomplete. They are frustrating to biocultural anthropologists because they fail to consider critical issues, such as raw-ingredient sourcing, and the local to global implications, for food producers and marketers, of the food industry's construction of globalised demand for such standardised fare. Their studies also ignore the nutritional dimension; for example, quite simply whether fatty and salty fast food is good for consumers who might otherwise eat healthier, more nutritionally balanced diets. From an ecological perspective, McDonald's' demand for a standard variety of potato, optimal for rendering the largest quantities of standard fries, has affected local agricultural economies, societies and potato biodiversity. Although not all ethnographic studies examining the impacts of globalisation can deal with every dimension of local change, they are part of the context and in a book about research methods these points should be noted.

Similarly, North American anthropologists increasingly study cuisine as a window not only on to culinary culture, but on to local or national political economy and 'identity' as well. Many accounts are examples of what Marcus and Fischer (1986) term 'experimental ethnography', in that they make the role of the ethnographer central to the *problematique* and exposition, and also blend into the analysis evidence from the print media, advertising, television and film. Wilk (1999) begins by comparing two meals: the first (in 1973) consisted of store-bought, imported canned goods, the second (in 1990) an array of fresh foods prepared from local ingredients. Both had been offered to Wilk, the anthropologist, as examples of prized local 'Belizean food', and their contrast provides Wilk with an entry point for tracing the changing symbolism of local foods (including edible rodent) in Belizean national politics. This analysis, which looks at the many elements of different national cuisines that enter into the newly created Belizean national food identity, addresses the political-economic and ecological dimensions of dietary sourcing, but once again leaves

out nutrition. The data collection and analysis are with one exception qualitative, and consist of field observations, interviews, descriptions of food and its
political uses garnered from print and film media. In the one quantitative survey
component, 389 Belizean respondents were asked to rate twenty-one main
course dishes (eight of which were judged to be Belizean) on a 4-point scale
from 'love' to 'hate'. Wilk found that there was no clear hierarchical set of
preferences for Belizean or non-Belizean dishes: 'The responses were striking
in their lack of clear order or hierarchy; tastes did not cluster together, nor did
they help disaggregate the population by class or education.' He notes that 'all
showed a high degree of agreement in their preferences for basic nationalised
dishes like rice and beans or tamales. Fourty-one percent of high school students,
for example, volunteered rice and beans with stewed chicken as their favorite
dish on an open-ended question.' (Wilk 1999, p252). On the basis of these
responses, the author concluded that a dish such as rice and beans with stewed
chicken is a preferred national dish across ethnic, age and income groups. This
class-neutral finding, however, reveals nothing about who had access to this
dish or how often, i.e. whether all those who prefer to eat this national dish in
fact could do so. Responses to follow-up questions, such as how often one
would like to eat this dish (numbers of times per week or month) and how
often one in fact does consume it, and the reasons for any discrepancies (e.g.
no opportunity to prepare it or too expensive) might have produced very interesting additional information on class differences in eating habits. Nor is there
any additional nutritional information in this 'real Belizean food' study.

Other studies of food and identity, again in Latin America, zero in on the
ways foods and their social and political distribution express indigenous and
also gendered identities. In Bolivia, for example, Healy and Paulson (2000: 15)
report how:

> Indigenous organizations such as the Andean *ayllu* and the Guarani
> *mburuvicha* have been revitalized as organizational forms for imple-
> menting rural development programmes, while women's and indigenous
> material culture has also been revalued leading to increased prestige,
> higher prices and export possibilities for quinua and for alpaca fiber and
> llama meat; consolidation of South America's first organic chocolate
> industry using organizational dynamics reflecting democratic Andean
> norms...

The authors indicate that social scientists studying in the Andes and Amazonian regions have both learned from and contributed to their efforts to revitalise
and sustain indigenous identity through the production and modern marketing of indigenous foods. Such anthropological exercises involve both research
and action, as anthropologists engage their subjects in strengthening indigenous resources, including indigenous livestock and tubers, as elements of
local, regional and national political economy and cultural identities (Healy
2001).

Food and its symbolism, when used politically, may also contribute to re-vitalising identities (see also MacClancy this volume). Firstly, in Bolivia, one politically and emotionally charged image is that of the traditional female, in local terms, the *chola*, who is a market woman, agriculturalist, *chichera* (associated with manufacture and distribution of maize beer (*chiche*) and establishments where it is consumed) and anchor of the household and regional economies (Albro 2000). Secondly, food may be given as a political gift, which is interpreted as in keeping with traditional norms of redistribution and exchange. Politicians exchange basic foodstuffs for political capital (the promise of household votes), and these contributions apparently are large enough to form part of subsistence calculations in some households. As another kind of political gift, food also figures in self-help 'food for work' programmes. These are variously interpreted either as part of the arsenal of anti-poverty programmes of a municipality, which claims to be an analogue to ancient communal work programmes, or as part of the social-welfare programmes of international NGOs, which put women (as embodiments of household well-being) at the centre of distribution networks and nutritional impacts. A third element for charting the connections of food to political identity is the location and role of the *chicheria* (the place where maize beer is sold and consumed), which serves as a centre for sociability and as a political cooking pot. A fourth element is the timing, elaboration and contents of periodic festivals, which link communities as well as individuals and households within them.

Each of these food-related components of social and political life constructs cultural identity, but also provides a nutritional context, and so attention should be given to such factors by the researcher into the anthropology of food. To complete a biocultural analysis, however, one needs to know more about how well the *chola* is able to get by on (scarce) resources, which usually include her time and work efforts, as well as the material and monetary resources that she commands. What is the actual value of food that politicians 'gift' and what is its timing? Is the *chicheria* a context where males replete their caloric intake and meet other psychological needs or demands, but at devastating cost to the well-being of their women and children? Are the timings and workings of periodic festivals such that they employ and feed economically disadvantaged individuals or households at critical times in an annual cycle that includes periods of dearth? Without going overboard in the direction of cultural materialism, which, as Mary Douglas in *Purity and Danger* (1966) rightly criticises, over-emphasises hygiene and medical health, it should be possible to connect political-economic observations and analysis to nutritional measures of biological well-being, and so to expand the analysis. This has been the most important goal of biocultural anthropology, at least since the 1980s (see Goodman and Leatherman 1998), and is relevant to the planning of fieldwork in 'food and identity'.

Moreover, there are ways to collect dietary information so that it can provide both cultural and biological insights, even without additional anthropometry or laboratory studies. In the brief study below I use Mexican data assembled originally for a UNAM (Mexican National Autonomous University) Quincentennial culinary symposium on the 'Encounter of 1492' to sketch what kinds of information and analysis might constitute such a biocultural study of identity.

## Indigenous Foods and Identity in Southern Mexico

Ask someone what comes to mind when they think of Oaxaca, Mexico and they likely will respond: 'the food!' Then they are likely to wax rhapsodic about the *mole* (a complex chilli and chocolate-based sauce served with turkey or chicken), *mescals* (distilled century-plant liquor) and whipped hot chocolate, all of which in the local culinary cultures are not only components of ritual meals, but also representative of the fusion of Spanish and indigenous elements which entered into folk Catholic customs during the colonial period. A visitor fortunate enough to arrive at the end of October through the beginning of November, the All Saints Day/All Souls Day season, would also observe, in a Geertzian sense, that this end-of-the-rainy-season harvest time is a busy economic and full ritual time, as special foods (chocolate, ground chilli for *mole*, rich decorated breads) are prepared for consumption and exchange across households.

The more distinctive elements of the contemporary food cultures in the towns and city of Oaxaca, in the southern highlands of Mexico, provide living testimony to the successful fusion of indigenous and European ideas and materials. In the 1930s, anthropologists would probably have explored which were indigenous and which were Hispanicised elements of the cuisine. By the end of the twentieth century, this question became perhaps less interesting than how local indigenous people adapted European grains, fats, animals, fruits, vegetables and herbs, sweets and distillation technology into their culinary calendar round. Messer (1996) noted that many of the ritual foods, such as breads, sweets and sweetened chocolate, and some of the spices incorporated into *mole*, were high status foods of Hispanic origin, as were meat from pigs and the occasional cow, sheep or goat. These were all expensive festival foods. But alongside these introductions, the everyday indigenous diet – maize, beans, squash, avocados and greens – remained basically the same (at least up to contemporary times of greater market food purchases). Snack foods, such as fruits, and also garden vegetables and spices were an interchangeable mix of plants of New and Old World origin. The more interesting questions for a nutritional anthropologist appeared to be the intracultural variations in the diet, and also whether the diet, as it underwent change, remained nutritionally adequate. To answer these questions, it is convenient to frame culinary observations in terms of food systems, dietary structure and principles of nutritional sufficiency, and then discuss how particular versions of the local diet relate to cultural identity.

# Food Systems, Dietary Structure and Nutrition in a Mexican Town

Traditional subsistence diets are constructed from the foods that are available in the surrounding environment plus any non-local foods (such as salt and chillies) that are necessary and affordable beyond that. There are also additional cultural principles, such as customary rules of what species are edible, inedible or preferred, local notions of a healthy, balanced diet and additional cultural factors, such as the religious calendar. All these features need to be observed by the researcher.

The setting for this example is a bilingual town located in the Valley of Oaxaca, in the southern highlands of Mexico, circa 1980. Located about an hour from the state capital, and connected to it by an hourly bus, the town is economically tied to the tourist economy and has been experiencing a decline in home-food production, which traditionally meant maize, beans and squash, plus some houseyard fruits and vegetables, a few poultry, and possibly a pig or a few goats. In this cultural setting most households purchase most of their foods in the marketplace. But there is still a small proportion of folk who gain their living from the land, and a larger proportion of households which still home-produce some of their maize.

## Dietary Rounds, Social Relations and Social Status

In this locality, most food comes from cultivated sources, and in the traditional diet, more than half the food energy is derived from maize; complementary protein comes from beans (grown with maize) plus garnishes of meat, cheese and eggs, while micronutrients are supplied by vitamin- and mineral-rich salsas, greens and fruits. Traditionally, people participated in a seasonal dietary pattern that followed the agricultural year with home-produced products supplemented by marketed goods. Dovetailing with this was a festival cycle: All Saints Day/All Souls Day marking the end of the harvest season, followed by Christmas and New Year's Day, then the patron saint's festival at the end of January, Holy Week and Easter, and community saints' festivals (*mayordomos*) scattered across the agricultural rainy-season months and leading up to the next All Saints Day/All Souls Day. In addition to this annual festival cycle, every year there would also be a number of multiday wedding celebrations, baptisms, confirmations and funerals, all of which involved the preparation of large quantities of food. These ritual meals feed not only the immediate guests, but also extensive circles of kin, fictive kin and neighbours, as all festival foods are widely distributed and redistributed. In traditional communities, the poorer members assisted at these festivals, which enabled them to eat a diversity of high quality foods for days at a time. A colleague, who worked in another nearby town, estimated that the consumption of nutrient dense sauces, animal protein and concentrated calories at these festivals could have fed participants one day in ten over the course of a year (Diskin 1978). Participation in such festival food preparation and consumption therefore embodies an important part of their individual and community biocultural identity, and researchers should pay attention to the social and biological consequences of such participation.

There are also additional ways to understand the way food marks distinctive and sometimes shifting cultural identities. With respect to subsistence, it is possible to document and describe patterns of wild plant collecting, as this supplements agricultural and market sources of food (see also Szabó this volume). The things to study are: what are the species, who gathers, prepares and consumes them, whether people want to eat them, and what does consumption of wild greens or other foraged foods signify about one's identity? In the case at hand, knowledge of wild plant resources is disappearing because most individuals are involved in market-based economic activities and go to the market for their food. Only the old timers have a good working knowledge of indigenous 'starvation' foods that were last consumed in some quantity during the most recent famine, which was 1915–1916, the period of privation surrounding the Mexican Revolution. Wild fruits and tubers, still locatable on the hillsides, are classified not as 'edible food' but as items that some individuals (such as shepherd boys, 'who will eat anything') eat when hiking through the hills. To understand the ways these foods enter into economic and social identities, a researcher ideally should forage for these items with individuals of different economic and occupational backgrounds, and also interview women and men of different ages to compare their knowledge of plant species, their classifications (see also Szabó this volume) and find out who (if anyone) eats them. As a special case, the eating of insect foods, such as maguey worm or toasted grasshopper, may communicate social and income class, as these items may be consumed more by those of low-income status who cannot afford to buy meat, even poultry, or by those of high-income status, who express an elite Mexican interest in traditional foods and culinary history.

Culinary descriptions can be derived from household, field and market interviews and observations, and then compared with additional sources. In Latin America, these additional resources include archaeological evidence of natural-resource use, ethnohistorical sources, including dual-language word lists, dictionaries and the royal *Relaciones Geográficos* that provide a basic inventory of resources by town. In many countries, there has also been considerable interest in the indigenous food heritage on the part of botanists, natural-resource managers, agricultural experts and public-health providers. Universities, herbaria and social-security health departments all provide potential interest groups for ethnobotanical research as well as sets of comparative data on edible food plants.

With respect to edible greens, people also recognise different community culinary customs. Prior to the early 1970s, some proportion of the local males travelled regularly with pack animals to more isolated ethnic areas, where they spent days and nights, and also learned the local foods. On the road, they observed food habits different from their own, for example, that in these distant settlements certain species of greens, that they customarily classified as 'inedible' and never ate at home, were cooked and eaten with squash leaves, and eaten, moreover, without ill effect. These men could make the distinction between culinary cultures, and also contextualise species that were biologically versus culturally 'edible'. Which greens one considered to be edible was thus a point of community cultural identity.

At another level, cultural knowledge and the practice of eating distinctive combinations of indigenous greens was disappearing altogether with recent changes in livelihood and trade. Even at home, 'wild' greens were low-status foods and not preferred. One low-income craftsman, whose household, out of economic necessity, still collected and consumed unsown amaranth greens from the fields, asserted that greens were only tasty, or real food, when there was plenty of fat (lard) to go with them, and, he said, 'when I have money I won't eat amaranth leaves (wild greens) any more'. However much nutritionists promoting green vegetable consumption might deplore such attitudes, such consumption preferences are part of cultural and socioeconomic identities. They can threaten good nutritional balance if these wild greens are not replaced in the diet by foods of comparable or better nutritional value. So, a researcher in nutrient intake must also take the time to study such cultural preferences.

Other elements of customary culinary cultures that distinguish one town from the next are the customary spicing of dishes (with garden or hillside herbs, as in the bean dishes mentioned above), and also general local preferences for sweetness, saltiness or piquancy. People distinguish between their own very piquant *moles* and the 'sweet' *mole* preparations of Oaxaca City and other towns, where cooks add sugar to offset the piquancy of the concentrated toasted ground chilli. Chocolate is customarily ground with sugar and cinnamon, occasionally with almonds but not with the vanilla characteristic of urban chocolate preparations. In this Mexican example, everyone takes their beverages very sweet, but recognises that individual and household preferences for degree of sweetness vary, and this variation is yet another distinctive feature of household culinary style and identity. Researchers into taste phenomena offer experimental protocols (see Simmen *et al.* this volume) to quantify sweetness perceptions and preferences, which can then be correlated with actual sucrose consumption and its (possibly damaging) nutritional and health consequences for individuals. For example, continual feeding of sweet beverages on demand to a toddler can reduce appetite for more nutrient dense foods, lower food intake and precipitate malnutrition (Messer 1986).

People also mark their political-economic and social identities by the frequencies with which they eat certain foods and by their manners of preparation. The substitution of bland breads for tortillas, and of pastas and rice for beans, may add variety to the diet, but their consumption threatens the traditional foundations of the food-based cultural identity, which centres on maize, with complementary beans and squash. Researchers, therefore, should not only be concerned with the consumption patterns and preferences that they observe, but they should also gain an understanding of changes that occur.

## Ethnobotanical Studies: Changing Relationships Between Humans and Maize

The changing role of maize in the local diet and food system offers additional insights into the ways changing food systems influence cultural identities, especially gender roles. For instance, one should find out if maize is home pro-duced (sown, cultivated and harvested) so that the household has year-round supplies of its own superior local variety. If maize is not home produced, it is worth finding out if the household can afford to purchase local varieties, or if it is dependent on market supplies, or, if the household is very economically disadvantaged, whether it depends on inferior-quality government-subsidised supplies. Does a household make its own tortillas, and if so, who does the bulk of the work, and how does that influence a woman's other work and her social identity? If tortillas are not made at home, are they purchased from relatives or neighbours, in the marketplace, or in the mechanised tortilla shop, whose product is usually classified as inferior?

Removal of women from the household labour of making tortillas suggests major changes in the cultural roles of women, who used to devote much of their day to maize preparation. Daily they would get the maize, cook the kernels with crushed limestone, then wash the cooked kernels removing their outer skins. They would then trek with their buckets of maize to a local mill, where it was ground (replacing hours of grinding at home), then they would return home, where they handground the dough one final time on their stone quern. They would then form it into tortillas, which they cooked on a clay or metal griddle that was fired with corn cobs, or with dry bamboo and sticks that the women had had to gather in the hillsides. All of this maize-related activity was very time consuming, and the release of income-earning women from this labour widened a market opportunity for women who had no other source of livelihood other than to make and sell tortillas. Also, it later created a market for machine-made tortillas. Machine-made tortillas had not yet entered this population in quantity in the early 1980s and were still judged to be an infe-rior product, made from inferior non-local maize that was not properly cooked.

The rise of the cash economy and decline in maize agriculture also changed the cultural roles and values of males, whose traditional identity was with and in their *milpa*. Furthermore, for the community as a whole, the decline in maize agriculture and diet signified fundamental changes in symbolism and meaning. As is the case throughout Mesoamerica, maize is a plant of extraordinary cul-tural importance. In the indigenous vernacular, all parts of the maize plant serve either directly or indirectly as food. In local folklore, maize is the only plant discovered by indigenous cultural heroes and Catholic saints, who also

participate in its cultivation. Maize grains enter into indigenous curing cere-
monies for soul loss, for removal of warts and also for divination. In the
indigenous language, four colours (white, yellow, red, dark) and also speckled
maize are recognised and named. A four-colour classification scheme is cosmological, rather than strictly biological, because the ancient and present cos-
mology is based on a four-sided or four-cornered universe, and the selection
of these four colours is arbitrary (i.e. there are more than four hues). An interesting question for cultural continuities and indigenous identity is whether
respondents recognise the symbolism in current practice, or are aware of its
indigenous cosmological roots.

As suggested above, as people move away from home production and into
the marketplace, they eat diets that are less dependent upon maize as the
staple food. Although the calorie intake of traditional diets of subsistence
households was measured to be 70–80 percent from maize (Messer 1978),
richer diets contain more of their calories in non-staple foods and more bread,
rice and pasta are consumed as carbohydrates. One can observe the decline of
maize in the daily meal cycle. Traditionally households began the day with a
morning 'coffee' and first meal (*almuerzo*, which is translated 'lunch'), then ate
the main meal of the day in the afternoon, and finished with another 'coffee'
at the end of the day. The morning coffee and first meal were based on tortillas and lubricated with maize gruel. The afternoon meal was also based on
tortillas, and the evening repast was toasted tortillas dipped in weak coffee or
tea. Today this same round of meals might include coffee-flavoured sugar
water and bread as the morning coffee, more coffee with the first meal, soft
drinks with the main meal and bread with the closing coffee or tea. For either
the morning or the afternoon meals, bread might be substituted for tortillas.
Whereas people used to snack on tacos if they got hungry at other times in the
day, these snacks today are as likely to be sandwiches or crackers. In similar
fashion, households, that no longer grow most of their own beans to consume
as income in kind, now purchase potatoes, rice and pastas as cheaper and
equally filling substitutes. What does not seem to be disappearing, however, is
a continuing taste for piquant food: chilli peppers and salsas accompany non-
local and enriched diets as well as the basic diet.

In sum, to understand this total range of relationships between individuals,
households, communities and maize, warrants cross-disciplinary study and
cross-community comparisons. Where the identity of males is no longer linked
to their maize fields and that of females to their competence in feeding their
households with homeground tortillas, what replaces these gendered and community identities, and how is the nutrition affected?

## Ethnomedicine, Diet and Medicine

An additional nutritional or medical dimension affecting the classification and
consumption of food and cultural identity is that of humoral classification of

food, diet and medicine, and its implications for dietary balancing in nutrition and health (Messer 1981). Traditional societies the world over customarily classified their bodies and the elements, and the foods and medicines that humans ingested, in terms of hot/cold and wet/dry. These terms referred to intrinsic qualities rather than to actual temperature or moisture. Health-promoting behaviours aimed at achieving a balance of qualities, because imbalances were associated with illness. Traditional recipes, such as the preparation of 'hot' beef soup with 'cold' coriander leaf, the consumption of 'cold' water with 'hot' salt, or the alternation of 'hot' and 'cold' qualities of foods and meals across the days and weeks could be rationalised as health-promoting behaviour designed to maintain the balance of qualities. Illnesses, which were also diagnosed according to their hot and cold qualities, were treated by their opposites, as in the case of 'cold' stomach ache or diarrhoea, treated by 'hot' spearmint tea. Such classifications demonstrated the natural and cultural balance of the culinary world, and also provided the household diagnostician with a recipe for illness assessment and curing by the principle of opposites.

Although modern physicians have sometimes disparaged such customary practices, anthropological analyses show that such systems of dietary classification are able to accommodate new elements without distorting nutritional balance. These analyses also underline the cognitive virtues of having such cultural classifications as a way to manage the troubles of unexplained illness. People expect that dietary adjustments will accompany pharmaceutical remedies, and physicians can accommodate hot-cold beliefs and practices by taking them into account. They can then recommend adjustments in their regimen, such as that a particular medicine (that the patient might classify arbitrarily as 'hot') be taken with a juice (that the patient classifies as 'cold'). A few simple questions can sort out these requirements and adjustments and meet cognitive as well as pharmacological requirements of a successful cure.

From an 'identity' perspective, the particulars of such beliefs and practices, including who holds them, uses them, passes them on from generation to generation, the structure and logic, as well as the intracultural variation, are essential parts of the ethnographic research of nutritional and medical anthropology. In the simplest and last analysis, a relevant cultural-identity question is whether in the contexts of modern lifestyles, diets and medicines, such beliefs and practices persist at all, and if not, what replaces them.

## Note

In Mexico, there has been considerable interest in indigenous food heritage on the part of the National Herbarium faculty, located at UNAM, and the national agricultural college and school of graduate studies. All provide an interest group for ethnobotanical research as well as sets of comparative data on edible food plants.

# References

Albro, R. (2000) The Populist *Chola*: Cultural Mediation and the Political Imagination in Quillacollo, Bolivia, *Journal of Latin American Anthropology*, 5(2): 30–88.

Diskin, M. (1978) Discussion in Symposium on Mexican Food System, paper presented at the 77th Annual Meeting of the American Anthropological Association, Los Angeles, California.

Douglas, M. (1966) *Purity and Danger*, Routledge Kegan Paul, London.

Goodman, A.L. and Leatherman, T.L. (1998) (eds.) *Building a New Biocultural Synthesis: political economic perspectives on human biology*, University of Michigan Press, Ann Arbor.

Healy, K. (2001) *Llamas, Weavings, and Organic Chocolate: Multi-cultural Grassroots Development in the Andes and Amazon of Bolivia*, Notre Dame Press, South Bend, Indiana.

Healy, K. and S. Paulson (2000) Introduction: Political Economies of Identity in Bolivia, 1952–1998, *Journal of Latin American Studies*, 5(2): 2–29.

Marcus, G. and M. Fischer (1986) *Anthropology as Cultural Critique: An Experimental Moment in the Human Sciences*, University of Chicago Press, Chicago.

Messer, E. (1978) *Zapotec Plant Knowledge: Classification, Uses, and Communication About Plants in the Valley of Oaxaca, Mexico*, Memoirs of the University of Michigan Museum of Anthropology Number 10, Part 2, Michigan.

Messer, E. (1981) Hot-Cold Classification: Theoretical and Practical Implications of a Mexican Study. *Social Science and Medicine*, 158: 133–145.

Messer, E. (1984) Anthropological Perspectives on Diet. *Annual Review of Anthropology*, 13: 205–49.

Messer, E. (1986) Some Like It Sweet: Estimating Sweetness Preferences and Sucrose Intakes from Ethnographic and Experimental Data, *American Anthropologist*, 88: 637–647.

Messer, E. (1996) Zapotec Foodplants: The Encounter of Two Worlds. In Long, J. (ed.) *Conquista y Comida. Consecuencias del Encuentro de Dos Mundos*, National University of Mexico (UNAM), Mexico City: 30–38 (in Spanish).

Watson, J. (1997) (ed.) *Golden Arches East: McDonald's in East Asia*, Stanford University Press, Palo Alto.

Wilk, R.R. (1999) 'Real Belizean Food': Building Local Identity in the Transnational Caribbean, *American Anthropologist*, 101(2): 24–255.

# EPILOGUE
## SOME FINAL HINTS

*Helen Macbeth* and *Jeremy MacClancy*

This book opened with a discussion of the many sub-disciplines of anthropology and the many perspectives on human food. However, the message that we have also conveyed is that new researchers need not include *all* the perspectives nor master *all* of the techniques discussed. Our intention is that, through a greater appreciation of the diverse methods for researching human food, researchers can approach their chosen topic as fully as possible.

### Defining the Topic

Whether, at the outset, each researcher has only a very general idea of the topic to be studied or a clearly identified enthusiasm, an essential task will be to carry out as thorough a search of existing literature as possible. Since that literature may be dispersed across different disciplines, the invention of electronic search engines has made that task much, much easier. Researchers, however, still need to check the original texts. They should not be content with abstracts or summaries available through some search engines, as these can be misleading. Where possible, discussions with specialists familiar with the literature and/or with the society or population to be studied are extremely useful. Researchers would then be in a better position to identify more precisely the topic or question that their research will attempt to address. Selection of appropriate research methods depends, of course, on defining the problem to be studied. We hope that students and researchers who reach the point of deciding how to carry out their research will find the contributions in this book useful.

## Defining the Study Population

Traditionally, the many sub-disciplines of anthropology are concerned with humans in groups, 'communities', 'societies' or 'populations' (for a discussion of these terms see Layton 2002). However, the definition of how individuals are grouped within any population tends to have many perspectives, viewed both by those inside and by those outside of the group (Chapman 1993). Researchers are, therefore, advised to take considerable care in identifying, and defending their definition of, the group or groups that they intend to study, whether on local, social or biological bases. What is more, it is possible that their research into food habits will itself reveal interesting divisions within the population they have chosen to study. So, researchers should always be alert to within-population diversity.

## Ethics Approval

Since anthropological studies are studies on humans, a researcher should find out the processes of 'ethics review' required by their institution, by the funding agency or by the population to be studied. Many funding bodies will not provide finance for research on humans until there is proof of appropriate ethics approval. Most professional organisations have adopted a code of practice for ethical research, as have many funding bodies, research institutes and universities. Some of the principles are also supported by legislation in many countries, for example in the United Kingdom by the Data Protection Act, the Human Rights Act, the Race Relations Act, etc. Researchers should bear in mind the dignity, rights, safety and well-being of participants at all times. Ethical requirements today involve more than just the assurance that the research methods themselves do not cause the subjects harm. Researchers should also consider the possible impact of their findings on other individuals, groups and relationships, whether or not these findings are widely disseminated.

Researchers also need to ensure that subjects are fully informed about the study before they agree to take part, including what it will involve for them and how any information they give will be used. Their consent should be obtained before the start and reconfirmed as necessary throughout the study. In the United Kingdom and many other countries there are legal requirements with regard to personal information entered on to any computer. Data entered on to computer without any personal details and in no way attributable to any individual have traditionally been considered an exception, and generally it is then acceptable to publish results in terms of populations and subgroupings of the population(s) studied. However, this lack of personal details also reduces the information that may be highly relevant in anthropological analysis. Furthermore, consent must be gained before publication either of material concerning any one individual or of an anonymous quotation, even when the person concerned is not identified. Potential researchers should consider these ethical issues carefully while planning their research. If part way through their research they introduce activities or aspects that do not comply with the original consent of the subjects, further consent should be sought. This is necessary even at a late stage in the research, but prior to the dissemination of results which include the new aspects. Many universities and research institutes now have an 'Ethics Committee', which reviews applications for ethics approval. It is up to the researcher to find out what their requirements are, and how to make the appropriate application.

## Publication

Research should not be considered complete until it is disseminated. As pointed out by Garine (Chapter 1) biologists tend to feel greater urgency about the publication of their results than social anthropologists do, and this is to some extent related to the nature of their material and demonstration of its originality. Publication may be in academic journals or books, or through the increasing electronic means of dissemination. Publication of papers on a cross-disciplinary topic in journals, however, is far from straightforward. Journals which openly welcome interdisciplinary papers have been rare, although they do exist and are increasing. Most academic journals are specialist journals directed at readers from specific traditional disciplines. Yet, this need not be a disadvantage if authors of interdisciplinary research are prepared to angle the prime perspective of each paper, and the style in which it is written, to the requirements of the journal approached and of that discipline. Such flexibility in style may ultimately lead to a wider variety of papers being accepted in different journals and a broader dissemination of the research.

## Acknowledgements

We wish to thank the Chair of the University Research Ethics Committee, Oxford Brookes University, for helpful advice.

## References

Chapman, M.K. (ed.) (1993) *Social and Biological Aspects of Ethnicity*, Oxford University Press, Oxford.

Layton, R. (2002) Population, community and society in peasant societies. In Macbeth, H. and Collinson, P. (eds) *Human Population Dynamics: cross-disciplinary perspectives*, Cambridge University Press, Cambridge: 63–82.

# GLOSSARY

**activity diaries:** Records showing time allocated by individual subjects to different activities throughout the day for each day studied

**affective:** Related to sentiment or emotions

**age-set:** Group of people in same age cohort, a grouping that may have social recognition

**alimentary:** (i) Pertaining to food or nutrition; (ii) providing nutrition

**astringent:** A sharp taste sensation that makes mouth tissue feel puckered

**asymptote:** A mathematical term referring to a line that approaches a curve at infinite distance

**background radiation:** High energy ionising radiation naturally occurring in any specific environment

**basal metabolic rate (BMR):** The minimal rate at which energy is required by an organism to keep alive when resting

**bell-shaped curve:** A distribution curve shaped like a bell, usually describing a 'Gaussian' or 'normal' distribution

**bimodal distribution:** A distribution curve with two distinct peaks (modes), separated by a trough

**biomarker:** Something that can be used as a marker for the presence of a biological condition

**brain cortex (or cerebral cortex):** The outer layer of the brain

**caloric expenditure:** Energy output through activities and metabolism, measured in calories (see also energy expenditure)

**caloric intake:** The amount of energy derived from food and drink consumed, measured in calories (see also energy intake)

**carnivore:** An animal that feeds on animal substances

**chi-square analysis:** A statistical test based on comparing 'observed' and 'expected' data in a matrix

**cognitive:** Related to thought processes

**collectivism:** The political theory concerned with collective control and distribution of labour, produce and chattels

**composition tables:** (see food composition tables)

**consumer surveys:** Question and answer surveys designed to indicate the preferences that individuals use, as consumers, to make choices

**cross-disciplinary:** Pertaining to studies which cross the traditional boundaries between academic disciplines (see also interdisciplinary, multidisciplinary and pluridisciplinary)

**cuisine:** Food preparation, cooking; also a particular style of cooking food, recipes, etc., taken to be characteristic of some culture or locality

**culinary:** Pertaining to food preparation, cooking and methods of doing these

**diary methods:** Research methods based on records kept by respondents on a day-to-day basis; (in relation to diet, the estimation of quantities may use general household units)

**dichotomous questions:** Questions with only two options for answers, e.g. 'yes'/'no', 'agree'/'disagree'.

**dietary recall:** Dietary information based on memory of a previous day's, week's, month's or year's dietary intake (see also recall methods, retrospective questionnaires)

**direct matrix ranking:** A method for grading and arranging in a rectangular, tabular form, with rows and columns, selected categories using quantitative values for these categories

**direct observation (of activities):** Observation *in situ* by the researcher, or assistant, of activities while they take place

**discourse:** (i) Style of an argument or particular approach to a certain problem or topic; (ii) the terms used and the logic underpinning the argument or the particular approach

**discursive logic:** The logic of a discourse

**doubly-labelled water method:** A technique using the turnover of deuterium ($^2$H) and oxygen 18 ($^{18}$O) in order to estimate the amount of carbon dioxide produced during a time period

**Douglas bag:** An instrument for collecting and measuring exhaled air

**duplicate analysis method** (in relation to food intake)**:** A method whereby all food and drink consumed are weighed and measured, and duplicate, weighed samples are then chemically analysed, from which nutrients can be calculated

**emic:** The point of view of locals, or other 'insiders', and the terms within which it is expressed; as opposed to etic (see etic)

**energy balance:** The difference, positive or negative, between energy intake and energy expenditure

**energy expenditure:** The output of energy spent on activities and metabolism, usually measured in kilocalories or kilojoules (see also caloric expenditure)

**energy intake:** The amount of energy derived from food and drink consumed, external warmth, etc., usually measured in kilocalories or kilojoules (see also caloric intake)

**ethnobotany:** (see Szabó, Chapter Two)

**ethnocentric:** Viewing and evaluating the world from the point of view of one's own ethnic group

**ethnographic:** Pertaining to ethnography (see ethnography)

**ethnography:** A written account of a human social group

**ethnomycology:** The study of traditional cultural concepts about, and names for, fungi

**etic:** The point of view of the observer, or other 'outsiders', and the terms within which it is expressed; as opposed to emic (see emic)

**factorial method** (re. energy expenditure): A method that integrates the caloric costs of activities over a specific period of time, the duration of which is determined in a variety of ways

**field journal:** A diary or notebook, which a researcher maintains daily to note down observations and data while doing fieldwork

**flex heart rate:** A method that uses continuous minute-by-minute heart rate records as a measure (rather than average heart rate)

**folklore:** Cultural, usually oral, traditions of people, especially the rural peasantry of Europe and North America

**food composition tables:** Analytic tables indicating the energy and nutrient contents of food items

**food intake frequency:** The number of times per unit time that particular food items or classes of food items are consumed

**food inventory:** An inventory of foods, either consumed by an individual or group or found in a particular place like a store cupboard

**food system:** The holistic description of the interrelationship between (a) the ecological and market availabilities of foods; and (b) the sociocultural classifications of foods as 'edible' or 'inedible' and their rankings as 'preferred' or 'less preferred' foods, as well as the rules for distribution; and (c) the nutritional and medical consequences of particular cultural consumption patterns, including patterns of food sharing

**food tables:** (see food composition tables)

**food table error:** Error due to inaccurate use of food composition tables where, for example, the food item is not exactly comparable to that in the table

**French paradox:** a seeming paradox in some regions of France where there is high consumption of dairy fat and low mortality from coronary heart disease.

**gastronomic:** Pertaining to the art of good eating

**gustatory:** Pertaining to the sensations of taste on the tongue

**gusto-facial reflex:** When the face unconsciously shows the reaction to a taste

**health physicist:** A specialist who examines the impact of issues in 'physics', such as radiation, on human health and the rest of the environment

**heart rate monitoring:** A method that uses the relationship of the heart rate to oxygen uptake during each activity to provide information on the former

**hedonic:** Concerning the extent to which sensations are considered to be pleasant

**hedonic scale:** A scale on which the extent that something is pleasant or unpleasant can be marked

**hedonics:** The study of the extent to which sensations are considered to be pleasant

**herbalism:** (i) Originally an early phase in scientific botany; (ii) mixed scientific knowledge and folk beliefs in the use of plants for beneficial and curative purposes

**herbarium:** (i) Originally a group of books written by fifteenth century to eighteenth century herbalists; (ii) a collection of (usually dried) plants preserved in collections to aid scientific studies

**herbivore:** An animal that feeds on plants

**holistic approach:** An attempt to view the whole situation including all perspectives

**homonymy:** Words that are, or sound, the same yet have different meanings

**household:** (of people) The group of people who live together in one homestead, or eat together at one hearth, whether these people are related or not

**hydatid** or **hydatidiform cyst:** A form of cyst or tumour, usually internal

**iconic food symbols:** Foods that become major features for a particular community

**identity:** (see MacClancy, Chapter Five)

**indirect calorimetry:** Indirect method of measuring energy (usually expenditure)

**infraspecific:** Pertaining to the biological diversity of organisms within a species

**intake:**

> **caloric – :** The amount of calories derived from food and drink consumed
>
> **dietary – :** The amount of food and drink consumed in the diet
>
> **energy – :** The amount of energy derived from food and drink consumed, external warmth, etc., usually measured in kilocalories or kilojoules
>
> **food – :** The amount of food consumed
>
> **nutrient – :** The amount of nutrients derived from food and drink consumed

**interdisciplinary:** Pertaining to studies which involve the mutual interaction, and to some extent the integration, of perspectives from two to three academic disciplines (see also cross-disciplinary, multidisciplinary and pluridisciplinary)

**interview guide:** A list of suggested topics to discuss in an interview (an example is given in Chapter Three by Hubert)

**interviews:**

> **fully structured – :** Interviews that follow strictly a pre-planned structure and list of questions. These are useful where time is short and comparability of interviews essential. However, they risk being perceived as over-formal and less attractive by the informant
>
> **non-directed** or **open – :** Informal conversations on any relevant topic
>
> **open-ended – :** Discussions that are partly planned, but which wander wherever the conversation with the informant happens to lead
>
> **semi-directed – :** Discussions which cover predetermined topics but do not keep entirely to the pre-planned structure of interviewing
>
> **semi-structured – :** Interviews that follow a pre-planned list of questions, but are allowed to include further discussions that seem relevant

**macronutrients:** Substances required in the diet in relatively large proportions: carbohydrates, proteins, fats

**Mann Whitney rank order analysis:** A statistical method for comparing two sets of non-parametric data, using rank order

**mean physiological value** (re. nutrients): The average amount of a nutrient needed to be consumed per day to balance out the daily use or loss of that nutrient

**micronutrients:** Substances required in the diet in minute amounts: most vitamins and minerals

**millirem:** One thousandth of a rem (see rem); a unit used for measuring safe levels of radiation

**motion sensors:** Devices for quantifying motor activity

**modes of identification:** Means by which people claim or impose identity

**multidisciplinary:** Pertaining to studies which involve perspectives from more than two academic disciplines (see also cross-disciplinary, interdisciplinary and pluridisciplinary)

**multiple choice questions:** Questions for which several alternative answers are offered, one of which must be chosen

**nomenclature:** (i) A system for naming; (ii) science pertaining to naming

**NGO (Non-Governmental Organisation):** An organisation not controlled by a government

**non-parametric:** Describing data which do not fulfil the criteria of a 'normal' or 'Gaussian' distribution (see normal distribution)

**normal distribution:** A distribution of data, where the mean, the mode and the medium coincide at the top of a bell-shaped curve

**nutrient intake:** The amount of nutrients derived from food and drink consumed

**nutritional status:** The health status of an individual in relation to their nourishment

**olfactory:** Pertaining to the sense of smell

**omnivore:** An animal that feeds on both vegetable and animal substances

**paired comparisons:** Comparison of items in pairs

**parametric:** Describing data which fulfil the criteria of a 'normal' or 'Gaussian' distribution

**participant observation:** Research method where the fieldworker is supposed to participate in, as well as observing, the life of the local people that he or she is studying

**physiological value** (re. nutrients)**:** The amount of nutrient needed to be consumed in a day to balance out daily use or loss of that nutrient (see also mean physiological value)

**pile sorting:** A method based on grouping objects according to their overall similarity in the judgement of the subjects

**plant inventory:** An inventory of plants, their names and uses; an inventory of the plants used by a sufficiently large number of respondents in a research project

**pluridisciplinary:** Pertaining to studies which involve perspectives from more than one academic discipline (see also cross-disciplinary, interdisciplinary and multidisciplinary)

**precise weighing method** (re. food)**:** Method in which all ingredients for food to be cooked and all the food and drink to be consumed are weighed. Cooked foods are weighed again before serving. Waste is weighed and measured. (see also weighed inventory method). Food composition tables are then used to calculate nutrients consumed (see food composition tables)

**preference ranking:** Items are arranged by each respondent in order of their preference

**qualitative:** Pertaining to descriptive rather than numeric data

**quantitative:** Pertaining to numeric rather than descriptive data

**rad (radiation absorbed dose):** A unit used for measuring the energy absorbed from ionising radiation by person or material penetrated

**random spot checks:** Observations, usually of short duration, at randomly chosen times and places

**ranking:** Activity whereby respondents grade objects or the characteristics of objects on the basis of one particular criterion at a time

**recall methods:** Research methods where the respondent is asked to recall data from some previous time (most commonly the previous twenty-four hours), or in regard to habitual patterns (see also dietary recall, retrospective questionnaires)

**recipe error:** Error in food analysis arising through diversity in recipes or inaccurate attention to the recipe for a given food item or dish

**rem (roentgen equivalent man):** A unit used for measuring biological damage caused by radiation

**respiratory gases exchange:** The oxygen uptake and/or production of carbon dioxide during breathing

**retrospective questionnaires:** Question and answer surveys, the answers to which require recall of past events (see also dietary recall, recall methods)

**role holder:** Person in or enacting the role described

**scales:**

> **hedonic – :** A scale along which the extent that something is considered pleasant or unpleasant can be marked
>
> **4-point – :** A scale with four ranked options
>
> **5-point – :** A scale with five ranked options
>
> **9-point – :** A scale with nine ranked options
>
> **11-point – :** A scale with eleven ranked options

**scenario method:** A method of analysis based on imagining the most likely complete scenario from incomplete evidence

**similarity ranking:** The ranking of items according to respondents' views on their similarity

**species:** (see Szabó, Chapter Four)

**subject:** One who is the focus of a study; e.g. an informant, questionnaire respondent or person undergoing any other research test or observation

**symbolism:** The use of symbols to convey meaning

**synonymy:** The same, or almost the same item, described by different words

**systematics:** The practice of grouping units in a systematic way

**tastant:** A person tasting substances as a test (for example for research purposes)

**taste:**

> **supra-threshold – :** Taste sensations above the threshold of tasting the substance (see taste threshold below)

**– threshold:** The weakest level at which the taste of an item can be noticed

*taxon,* **(pl.** *taxa***):** A group (groups) of items, usually organic, associated together and given a particular name in classification

**taxonomy:** The science of classifying items (in biology, of classifying organisms)

**time and motion studies:** Studies of activities, usually of one focal individual or group in relation to times taken for each activity

**titration:** The method by which a stepwise series of dilutions is created

**toponym:** The name of a place, or a name derived from that of a place or region

**triadic comparisons:** Comparison of items in threes

**two-bottle test:** Test involving choices between two fluids in different bottles

**video recordings:** Audiovisual recordings taken by camcorder

**weighed inventory method:** An inventory involving the weighing of all food before it is consumed, plus waste and discarded food. Food composition tables are then used for the calculation of nutrients involved (see also precise weighing method)

# INDEX

CPSIA information can be obtained
at www.ICGtesting.com
Printed in the USA
JSHW021300110422
24809JS00007B/236